QUANTUM
PALEO

—•••—

DOUGLAS WILLEN, D.C.

QUANTUM PALEO

Copyright © 2012 Douglas Willen, D.C.

First Edition, June 2012

Published by Fight Productions, Inc.

Email: DrDoug@TheHealthFixer.com

www.TheHealthFixer.com

Trademarks—All brand names and product names referred to in this book are registered trademarks and unregistered trade names of their owners. There is no implied endorsement of any of them.

Disclaimers—This publication aims to provide accurate and reliable information regarding the subject matter covered. However, neither the publisher nor the author shall be liable for any loss of profit or any other commercial damages, including but not limited to special, incidental, consequential, or other damages.

ISBN 978-0-9850527-0-6

Library of Congress Control Number: 2012937264

Printed in the United States of America

For my wife Rachel, my son Max, and my daughter, Lily. You are my inspiration, my education, my context and my net for every leap I take.

Contents

Round 1

What are you fighting for?

"Two roads diverged in a wood, and I—
I took the one less traveled by,
And that has made all the difference."

Robert Frost

Quantum Paleo is a program about developing a mindset that will steer one towards transforming their health and body. Quantum Paleo is much more than a diet book; it is a tool that can catapult you to change your body, and take control of your future. The steps of change take time. Start off with the initial phase of 21 days. Then repeat as many rounds of 21 days as you need to reach your desired goal (round 1, round 2, etc.). Although the long-term plan takes time, the shift or catalyzing moment of transformation can happen in an instant.

I had a life-changing "shift" 25 years ago in Mumbai,

India. It was the day that I hatched out of my self-centered shell and realized that I wanted to impact the lives of others. The epiphany I experienced is still impacting me today. Changing the body is a process, but the mindset can change in an instant. When that moment occurs, you will need to choose between "Two roads". The first road is the most popular path. The second road is "the one less traveled by". The path you choose will make *"all the difference."*

Mumbai 1987

I was silently debating whether to quit or not, on the third day of a seven-day "Transformation Thru Laughter" workshop. Six hours per day of laughing. The 40+ participants were from at least two dozen countries. At 23 years old, I was probably the youngest person in the room by seven years. This was my eleventh month overseas, and my third month in India. The rain season in Mumbai typically starts in June, and with only two weeks left in May, we were pushing not only high temperatures but almost unbearable humidity, too.

Angry and apathetic, I was barely going through the motions at this point. I felt mislead by the class description. I assumed there would be some discussions, lectures, and instructions that would comprise the format of the workshop. However, on the first day the Israeli instructor told the group, "There will be absolutely no talking. You are not permitted to stand up and walk around. If you want to cross the 50-square-meter room, you will have to crawl, or shimmy on your butt." The floors were wall-to-wall cushioned material. There were no tables, chairs, or furniture in the room. We were not allowed to ask questions. The only break would be for lunch.

That's it. For seven days, we had to sit on the floor. Our job was to either laugh, try to laugh, or watch people laugh!

The first day, people started to clump together in little groups and begin to laugh. I was certain that people were faking it. I stayed off to the side, observing. I sat for hours by myself, analyzing and critiquing the whole process in my head. I quickly determined that everyone was full of shit and that this was a colossal waste of time. I passed the time playing little guessing games in my head. I was making assumptions about the participants and drawing conclusions about these people even though I never heard them speak. I started forming little "stories" about the people I was watching. I would observe the body language and familiarity that certain participants had with each other trying to deduce if they knew each other prior to registration. This escalated into even bigger judgments. *This person has enormous ears. That one looks conceited. This one looks rich. This one looks intelligent. That one looks lazy.* It went on and on in my head.

On the third day of the same routine, I was sitting alone, against the wall sulking and feeling sorry for myself. The instructor came over to me and whispered, "Quit!".

"What? … No! I'm not quitting!"

With a half laugh, half snort, "You already quit, so do us the favor and get the fuck out of here."

"This class is bullshit. I came here to learn about how laughter can transform someone. There is no talking, no discussion, no scientific evidence, no teaching … only a bunch of phony people pretending to laugh."

"Here you sit on the sidelines and pretend you are living your life. You do this in all areas of your life. You are a watcher, not a player. You have your opinions. You are cynical and ignorant, but worst of all, you feel sorry for yourself. Self-pity is ugly. Why did you register for this workshop?"

My arsenal of witty comebacks failed me. I just shrugged.

"You must always have something in your life worth fighting for! Transformation can happen in an instant. It is not in a book or a lecture. Make the decision and then jump in. Don't expect an invitation."

Then she added, "You have 10 seconds to decide, either 'jump in' or leave immediately."

She walked away without looking back.

Defiantly, I waited the whole 10 seconds, maybe 12.

Then I crawled over to a woman sitting by herself, cross-legged in a beautiful silk Sari. She was in her late 60's or older.

I moved towards her for two reasons. The instructor's words hit a deep chord in my heart. She was right. I always have such grandiose dreams of how I want my life to be, but I never take action. In life, I tend to sit off to the side like a pompous, self-righteous general on a hill, safely watching his soldiers battle below. I want to retreat the minute something becomes challenging. Typically, leaving a trail of excuses in my wake.

The second reason I selected her was she was the only person in the group that looked more pissed off than I did!

I was now sitting cross-legged across from her, an arm's length away. We were both scowling. She was old. Her face was hard with deep crevasse-like wrinkles. I forced myself to stare into her obsidian eyes. I flashed on a movie scene where the attorney sits across the thick glass partition from his death-row client.

We continued the staring contest. My judgmental mind started up again. It always did. *She is decidedly fat. I wonder if she has ever exercised in her entire life. How old is she? Her clothes and jewelry must have cost her a bundle. She probably drives a Mercedes.* My mind kept generating judgments and opinions, on and on.

She reached out with both hands and lifted my hands off my knees. She wrapped her warm hands around mine. I felt a jolt. My mind went blank. Silent. I looked at her for the first time without judgement. All of a sudden, I began to see her. I could see past the facade that my judging mind constructed.

Another minute elapsed. Our eyes locked. Our faces were expressionless. She started to laugh; real laughter. Immeasurable laughter! Her convulsive laughter was wagging her whole body.

I still couldn't laugh. I started to get angry again. *Why was she laughing? Was she laughing at me?*

Something happened.

I saw a flash of myself as an old man. Alone, bitter, paranoid, dirt poor and feeling sorry for myself. I was disappointed with my unfulfilled life. It was like a scene from a movie of the end of my life.

I found this vision to be funny! Suddenly, a smile crept up my face pushing out through my eyes.

The damn broke and my laughter started gushing out. My face, my body, my feet, every cell of my body seemed to be laughing. We both were laughing. Tears streaming. It wouldn't stop. We kept laughing, stopping and restarting. I felt cracked open and exposed, like when a glove gets turned inside out as its pulled off of a hand.

Her face melted in front of my eyes. Granite skin turned to satin. We laughed for more than ninety minutes. It built up and went quiet, followed by another wave of ridiculous laughter.

Time flew by, and then it was the end of the day's session. Remaining silent I helped the woman to her feet. Without speaking a word, we bowed to each other and went our separate ways.

The next day I was the first to arrive. People entered the room and selected a spot on the soft floor. The woman was absent; running late. Joining up with different clusters of people, I was laughing and feeling at ease. I was alive. I was playing. I was in it. Full out. I was happy for the first time in a long time.

After four hours we broke for lunch.

The instructor pulled me aside as I headed for the door. I thought she was going to comment on my shift in attitude.

Cutting to the point. "She died last night!"

"What?" I felt a sensation like a punch to my unsuspecting belly.

"The woman died about an hour after class. She sat down in the lobby, closed her eyes, and died with a smile on her face."

Numb. Utterly speechless. My body began to shake from the inside out.

"I wanted you to know," the instructor continued. "She had not seen her family for over twenty years. She was extremely wealthy but lived in solitude because her family hated her. She had no friends and was highly paranoid. She believed that everyone wanted to steal from her. She trusted no one. Hate and bitterness dominated her life. She knew she was dying. She came here to connect to one person before she died. She wanted to find laughter. Something that money couldn't buy. One person to "see" her, before she died. You! She found you! Thank you for fighting!"

She turned and walked away, without looking back.

I stood there and cried, and then it turned into a laugh, and then a cry-laugh-snot, all at the same time. I felt heartbroken and elated at the same time.

Twenty-five years later, I can still see it play out in my mind. That day changed me in so many ways. I continue to have my insecurities and my problems with prejudging people. I still have trouble "jumping in." I can lose my focus over and over again about "What I'm fighting for". I am determined to live my life "full out." I have a never-ending passion for helping people find their way. After learning how precious life is, I wanted to work with people and help them achieve changes in their life and health while they still have time. I also became interested in the connection between grief, regrets and anger and how they can deplete one's health and vitality.

This book is not a traditional diet book. Most diet books are more science than we need, and more complicated than is necessary. The book is uncomplicated by design. This book tells you what you need to know, and then challenges you to change your philosophy about how you view your body. You will lose weight. You can lose a lot of weight if you choose. Most of the popular diet books in the bookstores will yield positive results. *Quantum Paleo* is a book focused on the question, "*Why?*". Why do you need to change? Why should you eat this way? How do you want your life to be? If you changed your body, how would your health be different? Would people relate to you differently? How would your relationship with yourself change?

This is a book about having a shift. It's about transformation. It's about tapping into the core of change.

When you figure out, "What you are fighting for?" your whole life begins to transform.

This book is for anyone that still wants to fight. This is for the person that is ready to take a quantum leap in a new direction. It all starts with a single question.

What are you fighting for?

The Emperor's New Clothes

Remember the Hans Christian Andersen short tale, "The Emperor's New Clothes"? It reminds me of all my blind spots. It is hard to have a clear vision in certain areas of my life, especially regarding my own health. Coaching other people is a lot easier than coaching myself. Where are your blind spots? Is it in finances, relationships, health or how about your body weight?

The significance of this allegory will mean different things to different people. When I re-read the story recently it provoked some self-examination in the area of my own blind spots regarding my body weight, health and longevity. It is so much more than an elementary children's story. It is a story about vanity, blind obedience and arrogance. It confronts conforming to the status quo, pretentiousness, pomposity, social hypocrisy and collective denial.

A synopsis I found in Wikipedia will remind you of this tale.

"The Emperor's New Clothes is a short tale by Hans Christian Andersen, about An Emperor who cares for nothing but his own wardrobe. He hires two weavers who promise him the finest suit of clothes made from a fabric invisible to anyone who is unfit for his position or "just hopelessly stupid." The Emperor cannot see the cloth himself; but pretends that he can for fear of appearing unfit for his position or being thought of as stupid; his ministers do the same. When the swindlers report that the suit is finished, they dress him in mime and the Emperor then marches in procession before his subjects. A child in the crowd calls out that the "Emperor is wearing nothing at all" and others take up the cry. The Emperor cringes, suspecting the assertion is true, but holds himself up proudly and continues the procession."

You might think this is a stretch to use this story as an instrument to teach a health lesson. We could go in a lot of different directions, too. Collective denial could be compared to our small thinking about the food industry, why we defend refined-carbohydrate meals, and believing that low-fat diets prevent heart disease.

I have read this story a few times throughout my life, and this time it made me think about my own health. Believing what I want to be "the truth." Living under the veil of denial that makes me believe that my game plan is enough. Erroneously believing that my health regimen yields the results to overcome my own health weak points. The Emperor was only "duped" because he wanted to believe the con men. He pretended that his new clothes were magnificent, and real, because he was worried he would be perceived as being stupid or below his station. He wanted to look good on the outside, at all costs, even though the inside was tainted.

Did you ever have the feeling that you were not truly healthy, even though your blood test stated you were "normal"? The glowing test results are a sham because you know you are not truly healthy if you still need to lose weight, eat better and be consistent with your exercise. Do you feel comforted when your family tree is riddled with heart disease, diabetes, cancer, arthritis, obesity, depression and auto-immune diseases? It does not reassure me because I know I have work to do.

Jack Zipes, author of "Hans Christian Andersen: The Misunderstood Storyteller," suggests that "seeing" in the tale is presented as the courage of one's convictions. "Sight becomes insight, which, in turn, prompts action."

I love that line by Zipes: "Sight becomes insight, which, in turn, prompts action."

Over the past twenty-four months, my mom had a huge health scare with her heart. She had to have two stents inserted into her obstructed coronary arteries. My mother was prescribed a "cocktail" of medications. During this time, she had several medical procedures in a row. Thank goodness she recovered and her health appears to have stabilized. She has lost over twenty-five pounds and is keeping it off. She never misses a workout. Through diet and closely working with her healthcare team, she was able to lower her score on the Hemoglobin A1C test into a normal range. The Hemoglobin A1C test reflects your average blood sugar level for the past two to three months. The test gauges how well you are managing your diabetes and pre-diabetes.

My mom used this turning point to gain "insight", which in her case prompted action. She needed to get her diet under control. She dropped the grains and adopted a "Paleo" diet. A "Paleolithic" diet can be extremely supportive for the diabetic and pre-diabetic patient.

In February of 2010, I was thinking about my mom's plight, while I was laying on the couch weighing 205 pounds with the TV remote balanced on my roll of belly fat. My percent body fat was 27%. I was blind to my 'blindspot' (that's why we call them blind spots!). I was rehearsing in my mind all the things I could tell my mom to reclaim her health. I was ready to suggest health tips to get her back on track. I could not see that I was on a slippery downhill slope myself. I had sound advice for my mom and my patients, but I was in denial concerning my own health. I'm not talking about the river in Egypt (family joke: "Da Nile.")!

Before I could 'doctor' my mom, she called me on the phone and implored me to schedule my long overdue comprehensive physical examination. I agreed. My doctor ordered a bunch of tests. I completed a heart stress test, routine blood work, and a 64 Slice CT scan with Calcium Score. The tests revealed that I had early signs of plaque in my coronary arteries. I also had several markers that were out of the acceptable (normal) range in my lab work. My blood pressure was high normal. This means I was borderline hypertensive. I had occasional angina pain (heart muscle spasms) when I was working too many hours and not getting enough sleep. This put me in the ninetieth percentile of being at a heart risk for my current age. In other words, only 10% of men in my age bracket (45-50 years old) were at a greater risk (than me) of having a heart incident. If you knew me, you would have probably thought I looked in average shape for someone in their mid to late forties.

The test result were very upsetting. I was walking in my mom's footsteps. Actually, I was jogging in my mom's footsteps! I had the insight to know what needed to be done with my own health. I needed to take action.

I have always gone to the gym on a regular basis. My routine back then was three days per week of 10-12 minutes of cardio, followed by 20-30 minutes of weight training. This gave me the typical look of most of the 40–50 year-old men in my gym; a strong, stocky body with a fat gut!

It was a Thursday when I got the bad health report. I decided I would start first thing Monday morning. Do you ever do that? I had my big wake-up call. I decided what I was fighting for, and I was determined to transform my life. I was fighting to prevent a future heart attack. However, I needed a few more days to eat my favorite foods, polish off the ice cream in the freezer and drink some beer in front of ESPN one more time before I started on this monumental journey!

I gained two pounds over the weekend while I was mentally getting prepared for my transformation. A few things were different this time. I've said that before, too. I was scared. I felt it was possible that I could be facing a heart incident in the next five to ten years. I'm not ready to die, but I felt like I was slowly killing myself out of neglect. On top of that, I could not live with my blind spot anymore. I hated the part of myself that made excuses and was inauthentic. I wrote down a list of things I was fighting for on an index card and decided to read them every day. I also wrote down my first goal and deadline for weight loss.

190 pounds by 3/26/2010 (my birthday!)

I am fighting for:

My life.

My wife Rachel.

My children Max and Lily.

My parents.

Last but not least, I wanted to look good in a bathing suit!

My birthday would be in nineteen days. I decided to use my birthday as my end date for Round 1. On the morning of my birthday, I was nine pounds lighter. I was a little disappointed because I thought I could lose more weight during "Round One". I decided I would repeat another round.

My birthday was on a Friday. I needed to do another round to continue towards my goal weight. I would start Round 2 on Monday morning. I call this time between Rounds, the "Gap". The Gap can be challenging, so be careful! I didn't gain any weight over the "Gap" weekend. I worked too hard to allow myself to revert back to my old habits. I read and re-read my index card with my goals. This helped me stay focused. The Gap is a time to test the concept of moderation. The definition of moderation is, "the avoidance of excess or extremes especially in one's behavior." I want my patients to learn how to live and function with moderation, especially during times that they are not on a strict regimen. The *Quantum Paleo* program is only successful if one can learn how to live and stay healthy during their normal routine.

Therefore, I want people to practice living in the "Gap" successfully.

I totally changed my workouts for Round 1. I started doing three 45-minute spin classes per week, on Monday, Wednesday and Friday during my lunch break, along with 15 minutes of weight lifting. In addition, I would do an hour "boot camp" training exercise class on Tuesdays and Thursdays before work. It was not until 12 months later that I came across CrossFit as my preferred system of training. That story comes later in the book.

Nutritionally, I incorporated the *Quantum Paleo* program, of course!

My body started to visibly change. My belly was not protruding. My face gets thinner when I lose weight. My whole body was getting stronger. Round 2 was easier than Round 1. I knew my sugar cravings would disappear within 48-72 hours after I quit sugar. It only takes two to three days to get on track.

I lost another nine pounds for a total of eighteen pounds in two rounds. I was extremely happy with these results. One hundred eighty-nine pounds and holding. I went back to my doctor, and my cholesterol dropped from 286 to 194. My triglycerides dropped from 200 to 145. My LDL came down from 130 to 98. My HDL went up from 42 to 51. My blood pressure moved from 138/92 to 118/74.

My belly was flat, and I got my lab work into the normal range. My body fat percentage was now 19.5%. I maintained 189 pounds for the entire year pretty easily by just eating "Paleo."

I identify with the Emperor. I see what I want to see, and hear what I want to hear. Zipes also said in his book, "Hans Christian Andersen: The Misunderstood Story Teller," that "*seeing* is presented in the tale as the courage of one's convictions."

It takes courage to see oneself authentically. It takes courage to turn sight into insight and then have that launch us into taking action.

The child does not have the social filter that we wear as adults. The child in the story blurts out the obvious… "The Emperor is wearing nothing at all!"

Most of what we have to do to help ourselves is obvious. Regarding my own health, I am like the Emperor, believing what I want to believe. Conversely, in my practice I play the part of the child, blurting out the obvious. "You need to lose weight." "You need to stop eating like crap." "You should go Paleo!" "You need to make the following changes and start building your health, now!"

If you could parade your authentic, naked self in front of someone that had the clarity and vision of a child, what do you think they would tell you to do? What feedback would you give yourself? I'm not talking about medications. I'm talking about the plan of getting back on track and producing astonishing results.

Start with this profound life-changing question... *What are you fighting for?*

Write it down on an index card. Then write down a list of reasons that will motivate you. Now fold it in half and put it in your pocket. Read it every morning and every night. Don't wait, do it now!

Round 2

What is Paleo?

The word "Paleo" refers to the term "paleolithic" which was coined by the archaeologist, John Lubbock, in 1865. It derives from the Greek words *palaios* meaning "old" and *lithos* meaning "stone." It literally translates to "old age of the stone" or "old stone age." Today, "Paleo" is commonly referred to as a grain-free diet!

The Stone Age, or Paleolithic era, occurred from 10,000 to 2.5 million years ago. It was a time that our ancestors had to hunt and gather for their survival. Today we live in the agricultural era. We have been farming for approximately 10,000 years.

99.99% of your genetic blueprint was formed more than 10,000 years ago. In other words, your genetic makeup is virtually identical to your Paleolithic ancestors. Your genetic code was shaped over a period of millions of years. That means that certain foods and nutrients, the same ones your ancient biological ancestors consumed, are literally part of your biology today. Good health can be expected when you feed your body the foods to which it has genetically adapted. Conversely, when we feed our bodies food that we have not adapted to, dyspepsia, degeneration, and disease will follow.

In 1985, Dr. Boyd Eaton of Emory University in Atlanta, Georgia, wrote a landmark paper called "Paleolithic Nutrition", which was published in the prestigious New England Journal of Medicine. The basic premise of that report was that our genes determine our nutritional needs. For 2.5 million years, we ate what we could hunt and gather. Today we eat what looks good, tastes good and what is sold to us through multi-million dollar ad campaigns. The average American eats 150 pounds of sugars and sweeteners per year, and hundreds of pounds of grain.

The medical doctor, James Braly, and Ron Hoggan wrote a book called "Dangerous Grains." They share their research on how grains are linked to more than two hundred chronic illnesses and conditions, including Type 2 diabetes, cancer, heart disease, arthritis, autoimmune diseases, brain disorders, intestinal diseases, chronic pain, infertility and problematic pregnancies to name a few.

Our hunter and gatherer ancestors were tall, strong and had lean bodies. They survived on animal proteins like meat, fish and fowl. They had fruits and vegetables, nuts and seeds and good, healthy fats. Dairy and starches were only available intermittently. Livestock was not domesticated; therefore, they did not have access to milk producing animals on a regular basis. Root vegetables and assorted starches were not planted and farmed in the pre-agricultural era. Starches would fall under the category of items that could be "Gathered." Items that needed to be "hunted and gathered" were not always present on a consistent basis and were dependent on geographical location, seasons of the year, and numerous other variables that determined availability. Grains and sugar were not available during the Paleolithic Era. People of this time period did not have access to bread, pasta and other grain foods that are abundantly produced and consumed in today's world. Consequently, they did not suffer from the degenerative diseases of the modern world we live in today.

The Paleo way of eating is the only diet that closely matches the foods we should eat according to our genetic makeup and our evolutionary progress. The number one reason that "Paleo" works is that it matches the way we are designed to eat. I am seeing patients successfully "turn back the clock" to a time in their lives when they were not sick and tired all the

time. It is exciting to see people reclaim their health
and their ideal body weight.

What Are the Benefits of Going Paleo?

There are numerous benefits that one can expect by converting to a Paleo way of eating.

Six benefits that I see over and over again in my practice are listed below. Please share your results with me thru email which can be found at the back of the book. If you decide to share your results or experiences, I will place it on my website, and maybe include it in an upcoming book.

Six benefits of my specific *Quantum Paleo* program:

Weight loss:

You can expect to lose anywhere from 6–18 pounds in the first 21 days alone. I conducted a corporate team building *Quantum Paleo* event in the spring of 2011. It was set up as a group competition made up of two teams of 20 employees lasting only 21 days. One participant Bryan lost 26 pounds. A second male, Larry, lost 22 pounds. Dave lost 18 pounds, and six others experienced weight loss in the 13–16 pound range. Our top female competitor lost 15 pounds in just three weeks. We also had three other women lose from 9–12 pounds.

Health benefits:

The list of benefits is extensive. Most people will see positive results in their energy and stress levels within a few days. We also see improvement in such an array of health related areas affecting the immune, digestive, and musculoskeletal systems. Every person's results will vary. I would love to hear how this diet affects your health.

Sleep:

Removing refined carbohydrates, sugar, trans-fats, junk food, and chemicals from ones diet will result in better sleep.

Sex:

Getting healthy and returning to a body weight that makes you feel better about yourself will not only improve your libido, but will improve your partner's, too.

Longevity:

Eating the foods one is designed to eat will optimize health and longevity.

Strength and fitness:

The fittest athletes are eating a diet that closely resembles *Quantum Paleo*.

Grains: The good, the bad, and the ugly!

The plants that produce common grains such as wheat, rye, and barley have compounds such as lectins, gluten, and phytates that can damage your digestive tract and even trigger an autoimmune response.

Keywords that you need to know are gluten, celiac, lectin and phytates. I will cover these terms briefly in a "what you need to know" style, so that you can get started as quickly as possible.

Gluten:

According to Dorland's Medical Dictionary, Gluten (gloo'ten) is the protein of wheat and other grains that gives the dough its tough, elastic character. Gluten, found in wheat, rye and barley, is made up of the proteins gliadin and glutenin. The inability to digest gluten is becoming more prevalent according to researchers at the world famous Mayo Clinic.

Celiac:

Celiac disease, also called Celiac Sprue, is an autoimmune disorder of the small intestines that occurs in people of all ages. Around 1% of the population has Celiac disease. Symptoms include chronic diarrhea, failure to thrive (in children), and chronic fatigue. Celiac is thought to affect 1 out of every 133 people in the United States. When a person with this condition is exposed to gluten or other similar grain proteins in other grains, the immune system can cross-react with the small-bowel tissue causing an inflammatory reaction. This causes damage of the villi lining the small intestine. The intestinal villi are responsible for the body's ability to absorb nutrients. Therefore, vital nutrient uptake does not occur at a proper level, leading to malabsorption and even malnutrition issues.

Celiac disease is often difficult to diagnose. Many sufferers are not diagnosed for years. Some doctors believe that for every one patient diagnosed with celiac there are 30 people who go undiagnosed. It is also believed that many people have extreme difficulty digesting gluten but never manifest celiac disease. They have gluten intolerance and not the full-blown Celiac disease. Dr. Braly and Mr. Hoggan estimate that as many as 90 million Americans may have non-celiac gluten sensitivity. Both celiac disease and gluten intolerance are incurable, permanent conditions. The only known, effective treatment is abstaining from gluten and grains in general for the rest of one's life.

Lectins and Phytates:

Plants have a built in self-defense mechanism that they rely on for survival. For a plant to procreate, it must rely on other "outside" sources to spread its seeds. Sometimes it's the wind. Sometimes, birds and insects will aid in spreading the seeds. The plant cannot generate movement in order to spread its own seed to ensure its survival. Therefore, it has several "methods" to help the seed survive long enough for it to implant in soil at a distance from the original plant.

Grains produce compounds such as lectins and phytates. These are toxic substances that act as "anti-nutrients." An anti-nutrient literally prevents the body from absorbing certain vitamins and minerals by directly disrupting absorption. These compounds are poisonous to insects, birds and even humans, and make it very difficult for them to digest the entire seed or nut. The seed or nut will often be safely passed or defecated back into the earth.

Fruits are an exception because they are not "anti-nutrients" and don't pose the same danger as grains. When an animal eats fruit, the seeds will pass through and exit the body, too. This is a perfect design by nature. The seed survives because the seed is indigestible. Some animals have clearly adapted to grain consumption. Birds, rodents, and some insects can deal with the anti-nutrients. Humans, however, cannot.

Three Whites for 90 Days!

"80% of sick people would get well if they would eliminate dairy, wheat and sugar!" (Nancy Appleton from her book "Lick The Sugar Habit").

I love that quote, and I hate that quote.

I love it, because it is true.

I hate it, because it is true.

I love the three whites. Don't you? I hate telling my patients to cut out sugar, dairy, and flour. I hate telling a child to cut out the three whites. It works; sick people will get well. Chronically overweight people finally lose weight after years of failing.

Stan came to me about 10 years ago. Working as a restaurant chef, he needed his hands to function at a high level, but at the age of 44, he could not close his hands around a chef knife. Swelling and redness in the hands were his most aggravating symptoms. He could only partially bend his fingers. His knees, ankles, elbows and shoulders were also puffy and painful. His muscles in his back, neck, hips, buttocks, chest, legs and arms were constantly in pain. His family doctor gave him the diagnosis of arthritis and fibromyalgia.

I ran an IgG Food Sensitivity test as well as a test for Gluten. We also did some basic blood work. The test showed that he was reacting to grains, sugar and dairy. The gluten test was negative for Celiac, but it did indicate that he had a non-celiac gluten sensitivity. I told him to eliminate the three whites (all grains, dairy and sugar) for three months as a starting place. I put him on the *Quantum Paleo* program and he was optimistic about getting started.

Six weeks later he was pain free. The swelling and redness in his hands were back to normal. The fibromyalgia symptoms vanished. I kept him on a strict Paleo diet. When someone comes to my office and has serious health complaints, I am not lenient with the diet. They must do it 100%. Stan also lost 36 pounds in the 90 days. At the end of 90 days, Stan tried to reintroduce small amounts of bread and pasta into his diet. After a few hours, the pain and swelling returned. That convinced him to commit to the diet for the long haul.

If I'm ever stumped with how to help a patient with chronic health issues, I always take them off of grains, sugar and dairy. I have the patient clean up their diet. It works. I had a favorite professor in the Nutritional Sciences department at chiropractic school that would preach, "Start with the gut you can never go wrong."

If you have a chronic condition, especially if there

is an inflammatory component, then consider the possibility that food is a vital piece of the puzzle. Go off of the three whites and see what happens. It is essentially an "anti-inflammatory diet". I would be hard-pressed to come up with any disease that does not have an inflammatory component at some point during the presentation of that ailment. In other words, try cleaning up your diet and see where it leads.

The word "Paleo" is new for me. I only became aware of it about two years ago. I have been using a Hunter and Gatherer diet with my patients for 14 years. I would simply say, "Eliminate the three whites diet."

I have my patients eliminate the three whites for 90 days! I built a whole practice and career on that simple diet. Today everyone calls it Paleo, Primal, or Caveman! Who cares … "A rose by any other name would smell as sweet," (William Shakespeare).

Round 3

Quantum Paleo

What is *Quantum Paleo*? What does it mean? How is it different than what others are teaching, writing and blogging about concerning this subject.

That was a question my wife Rachel asked me when I started writing this book.

My point of view is what makes this program unique. This book is different because I come from a clinical background. I'm not a biochemist, anthropologist, or an elite athlete that has adopted this way of life.

I have put thousands of people on grain-free diets in the past 14 years. I have always used a "grain-free" program. Not because it was approaching the diet of our Paleolithic ancestors that most closely resembles what are bodies need today. I never heard of the term "Paleo" 14 years ago. I put people on 'grain-free' diets because "it got sick people well". Period. I also took people off of sugar and dairy too. It helped people reclaim their lost health.

Quantum Paleo is a book that includes the mindset that one needs to succeed. In my clinical experience, I have worked with so many people that need support on not only the "how to" but also the "why." *Quantum Paleo* drills down to the "soul" and "gut level" enabling people to make lasting changes.

I am excited to read the informative blogs and books on this subject. There is a whole world of 'Paleo People' in the Tweetosphere, too. I am even more excited to learn the reason that sick people get well on a grain-free diet: The Paleo way of eating is the only diet that closely matches what we can eat according to our genetic makeup and our evolutionary progress.

Great. We have an extraordinary diet. We even have a historical, anthropological and evolutionary reason to dial into this life-changing information. However, in the past fourteen years, I have run into a stonewall with patients about getting them to stick with the program long enough to see the results. If people do not have a crystal clear goal of *What they are fighting for*, they may not succeed. I eventually challenged my patients to incorporate the "why" into their goal setting. I found when patients wrote down on an index card their goals and answered the question of "What they were fighting for?", their results with chronic health conditions improved dramatically. Their resolve strengthened. The patients that did this basic exercise of writing down their goals tended to stick with the regimen long enough to see results.

Most of us do not choose to eat foods for the same reasons that our Paleolithic ancestors needed to survive. Our Paleolithic great aunts and uncles did not have the temptation of a breadbasket being put on the table every time they went to a restaurant. They did not have to stare down and resist a pizza or a birthday cake and overcome the urge to take a bite. I would be willing to bet if you offered a caveman a seat on your couch, an overstuffed sandwich, and a beer while you watched a Sunday afternoon football game, he probably would not turn you down.

We live during a time where many of us eat for pleasure. We emotionally select our foods without a single thought of life and death on our minds. The Paleolithic people probably experienced tremendous joy and emotional peaks eating their favorite foods of the day. The crucial difference was their primary concern was survival.

How does a person living today avoid all of the tempting, delicious foods and choose correctly? Are we supposed to avoid pizza for the rest of our lives? These are relevant and appropriate questions. My approach is to commit to a short schedule of time and get healthy as fast as possible. To do this, you must do the program with focus and intensity. Learn your body's nutritional needs to function and express health at its highest potential. Then make wise choices to achieve lasting health.

I have showed patients their blood work and supporting research that unquestioningly proves that they must change their diet. They have not been able to comply and stay the course even though they may succumb to the clutches of a symptom, condition or disease. Have you ever seen someone that had throat cancer surgery; their surgeon leaves a little hole in their windpipe to breathe and talk? I have seen throat cancer survivors remove their scarf and take a drag off their cigarette from the hole in their neck. They know they must quit. They still smoke through the hole in their windpipe. That person never had the mental shift that they needed to transform their life. I feel their healthcare is incomplete. They had a successful surgery. No one addressed the mindset. The person did not have a breakthrough on the soul level.

I have been face-to-face with people that need to change and want to change, but won't, and therefore don't!

My approach I call *Quantum Paleo*. This program not only addresses diet, exercise and lifestyle but it will help you uncover the beliefs and "hangups" that are holding you back. I also realize there may be people reading this book that do not need motivation or guidance. They get hooked on a new program and immediately gain momentum as the weeks go by. They are strong and athletic and have the willpower to make dramatic changes with very little guidance. If you are a person that succeeds easily then use this book as a quick guide book.

Most of my patients over the years need more than motivation, inspirational quotes, diet menus and weigh-ins to achieve success. I push my patients to dig down and find the limiting factor that is holding them back. They need to tap into something that is worth fighting for. It can only be found at a core level. When a patient finds the core reason to change it is extremely emotional. I have seen patients break out in tears. It needs to be something truly personal. It needs to touch their soul.

Next I pull on that thread and slowly unravel the fear, insecurity and regrets that accompany someone that has struggled with their health and bodies throughout their lives.

It takes a "Personal Leap" away from the current, traditional American way of eating in order to arrive at a new place of health and longevity. *Quantum Paleo* is the program that can take you there. *Quantum Paleo* is a program that has all the good "Paleo" stuff and addresses the emotional component at the deepest, core level.

Religiousness

The more I read about how Paleolithic eating is interpreted, the more confused I get. Some people write that to be "Paleo" you can not ever eat this or that. Some people loosely define the parameters of what constitutes a "Paleo" program while others are downright zealots!

The real extremists are almost to the point where they are ready to trade their jeans, T-shirt and credit cards for a loincloth and a spear. I call them "Paleo Evangelists".

I am not ready to give up a cup of ice cream every once in awhile. I also want to try my share of local and foreign beers throughout my life.

Beer, by the way, is not Paleo.

What a conundrum!

I also like chocolate. How about you?

I started with all this 'Paleo' stuff in my practice 14 years ago, trying to help sick people get well. The people calling for appointments were <u>not</u> healthy athletes, or CrossFit enthusiasts. They were not even healthy. They were chronically ill people and the word

'Paleo' was not even on my radar at the time.

I was taught by my nutrition professor, to take patients off of the three whites (dairy, sugar and grains) and 80% of them would get well.

At first, I did not believe that changing the way people eat could turn around their health picture. I was impressed at the results I witnessed after doing "the rounds" with him in his facility and talking directly to patients about their cases. I interviewed patients with serious health issues and heard dozens of stories of how getting off grains improved their health. The most impressive part was to see their objective blood tests support their subjective assessments of their symptoms.

What is the reason we should even give a crap about a Paleo type of diet? Is it because we secretly wish to live the simple, rustic lives of the hunters and gatherers? Some people do!

As a healthcare provider, I think the mass appeal is the remarkable health benefits that so many people are experiencing. The ability to maintain a lean, fit body, after years of failing miserably at so many popular diets is very appealing.

A few years ago, I heard the word "Paleo" for the first time. The 3-White Elimination diet that I was utilizing with my patients was essentially the same as today's Paleo diet. Whatever you call it, it gets results. If this is true ... then certain questions will inevitably arise.

"How strict do I have to be to get results?"

"Can I ever have a beer?"

"How about wine? Or a shot of tequila?"

"Pizza? Baguette? Tortilla? Crepe? Or how about Grandma's famous Chocolate ice-box-ladyfinger cake that has been passed down from generation to generation?

This is the point where I am sure I will get a lot of negative comments. I am not "the 100% guy" you may be looking for. My POV (point of view) is primarily as a healthcare provider. When I sit with a patient and evaluate their level of severity of symptoms and conditions, I will then recommend how intensely I want them to comply with the diet. If their overall health is compromised, I will recommend that they take this lifestyle program on at 100% for at least 90 days. No cheating. Full out! Then we will reevaluate how they are feeling at that point. All through this process I'm helping them make a lifelong transition to the "Paleo" mindset.

In my practice, I have the benefit of using a blood test called IgG Food Sensitivity Test. I have been using this test for almost 15 years. It will tell me how reactive dairy, grains, sugar and 96 different foods are to the body's ability to maintain health. If the patient completes the 90 days and the test shows they are clear on dairy, grains and sugar, I allow them to experiment with an ice cream or a beer. Whether the patient can maintain results after 90 days while eating an occasional "ice cream" depends on their ability to maintain homeostasis. That is my POV. I am 100% in the beginning. I try to work an occasional "ice cream" back into their lives.

The definition of the word "food" is: *Any nutritious substance that people or animals eat or drink, or that plants absorb, in order to maintain life and growth.*

The definition of the word "treat" is: *An event or item that is out of the ordinary and gives great pleasure*

According to this definition, ice cream is not "food". Ice cream is a treat. We don't need treats every day. It is the exception not the routine. This is crucially important. I will say it again. Ice cream, beer and bread are special treats, and should not be consumed every day. If your body can tolerate it occasionally, then enjoy it as a treat.

These days I work with a lot of healthy people. They are excited about adopting a new paradigm. Many are young, healthy, athletic, symptom-free people that already get the 'Paleo' mindset. With these folks we talk about balance.

To maintain an elite edge of vitality and health, you need to be on target with your diet. Period. Can you have the occasional beer night?

I want you to.

We are not living in the Paleolithic era. There are a lot of fun things to drink and eat. Staying in balance is the challenge.

Greg Glassman, the founder of CrossFit, said in an interview on the CrossFit Journal website conducted by Fast Company Magazine that, "many people are interacting with 'Paleo eating' in the same way that they follow religious precepts." Glassman goes on to say that many people get almost fanatical about every ingredient of food they touch and whether it is "Paleo" or "not Paleo." He gives an example of someone getting all upset because some parmesan cheese was on their food, and that parmesan was "not Paleo." The point he is making is that "Paleo" or "The Zone Diet" or any other diet that attracts the athlete and high performers of the world, are supporting the human potential. The diet you choose will either support or not support function and performance in the human body. Therefore, your focus should be on health and performance. It is not a competition about which person can go the longest time eating the perfect Paleo diet.

Greg Glassman concludes the segment by suggesting

a way to take "Paleo" up a notch is to control caloric intake and control portion sizes. I have always looked at combining both the basic 'Paleo' type of diet (proteins, vegetables, healthy fats, seeds and nuts, some starch, little fruit and no sugar) with an initial phase of calorie restriction.

The question then is why are you doing a Paleo diet anyway? Are you trying to get healthy? Are you trying to look good naked? Are you trying to have a diet that dovetails with your quest for improving athletic performance? These are all good reasons. Some people take it to an extreme level of trying to eat like an actual caveman and re-enact the true diet of the Paleolithic man. Everyone should be able to make their own choices.

Re-enacting the life of a caveman is not what I teach. I am a healthcare provider. My goal is getting results for my clients/patients. I feel the Paleo way of eating is superior to other approaches. Having said that, I explore with my patients the possibility of having some milk in their coffee. Having an occasional scoop of ice cream as a treat. We start with an initial stage of having zero grains, sugar and dairy.

How often can a patient veer into the realm of eating grains, sugar and dairy, and still maintain the highest level of health? It will be different for different people. Some people will learn that they can tolerate grains, sugar and dairy in trace amounts. Other people will learn that they can never have grains and maintain health. That's right. Never! I encourage my patients to be very strict and do this program at 100% for at least 21 days. Then the potential of the program can be experienced.

Is 90% Paleo okay? Is 99% better? Is 100% Paleo the only way to go?

I don't want to answer that question. We are all individuals on both the outside and inside. My advice is to dive-in, and do the program as written. Then see for yourself what works best. If your goal is keeping lean and fit, you might have a different percentage of compliance than someone that is living with a life-threatening bowel, digestive, or auto-immune disease.

Is Paleo Unhealthy?

"Are Paleo diets unhealthy?"

No!

I have been teaching and implementing a "Paleo" diet in my practice for over 14 years. I even led a Tuesday night ongoing group workshop/class for three years in NYC from 1999–2001. The program offered a "Paleo" diet with a herbal detox kit thrown on top. The program was based on a grain-free diet that included herbal supplements to cleanse the liver, gallbladder, blood tissue, kidneys and lymphatic system. I still use this *Paleo-Detox* with patients today.

Whenever I would teach the intro class, I would hear the same questions from students.

"Isn't it unhealthy to have zero grains in my diet?"

"What is left to eat?"

"If I eat only protein, vegetables, healthy fats, some fruit, seeds, nuts and plenty of water, won't that hurt me?"

"Maybe I should check with my "Regular Doctor" before I attempt this radical diet." By the way, does "Regular Doctor" mean that their bowel moves every day? And are they implying that mine does not? I digress.

I have had students in my class demand a refund after asking their "Regular Doctor" if eating this way was healthy. Their "Regular Doctor" told them, "grain-free diets are unhealthy, foolish and unscientific!"

My comment, "What a load of Wooly Mammoth crap!"

Let this sink in, the "Paleo" way of eating is the only diet that closely matches what we can eat according to our genetic makeup and our evolutionary progress. "Our genetic code determines our nutritional needs."

The following, is a short list of conditions that have **improved or resolved** in my practice over the last 14 years:

Malabsorption

Gastritis

Colitis

Chronic Diarrhea

Flatulence

Delayed Menarche

Liver Disease

Leaky gut syndrome

Impotence

Low Libido

Iron deficiency anemia

IBS

Kidney Disease

Heart Disease

Type 2 Diabetes

Grave's Disease

Alopecia

Nausea

Vomiting

Bloating

Ulcerative Colitis

Chronic Fatigue

Eczema

Edema

ADD/ADHD

Autism

Schizophrenia

Anxiety

Epilepsy

Failure to thrive

Gastrointestinal Bleeding

Cerebral Atrophy

Celiac Disease

Chest Pain

Cancer

Bladder Cancer

Brain Cancer

Prostate Cancer

Osteoporosis

Autoimmune Diseases

Lupus

Ataxia

Hyperthyroidism

Miscarriages

Amenorrhea

Arthritis

Fibromyalgia

Oral Cankers

Multiple Sclerosis

Trigeminal Neuritis

Myasthenia Gravis

Infertility

Still Births

Otitis Media

Pancreatitis

Depression

Osteomalacia

Rheumatoid Arthritis

Delayed Puberty

Eczema

Hives

Weight loss

PMS

Hemoglobin A1C improved scores

Psoriasis

Hypothyroidism

Vitiligo

This is not simply a list of conditions that I have read about in popular books. These are results from actual cases of people that I personally monitored that adopted a Paleo way of eating. Expect it will take 3–12 months to transform your health and body. Many people will be satisfied to have some of their chronic symptoms improve while others will find it shocking to have life-changing results.

What is possible?

The *Quantum Paleo* program can take you all the way back to reclaiming your body. Do not make it complicated. This book is about getting the vision to make a change. The main thing is to get started. Keep it simple.

"Whatever the mind can conceive and believe, the mind can achieve." - Dr. Napoleon Hill.

Round 4

The Challenge

I call this the **Challenge Section** because it will challenge you to think, plan, feel and take action. This is the section that separates my book from other Paleo books. I have worked with thousands of patients over the last 14 years. I have seen many people frustrated with their inability to lose weight and reclaim their health. Over time, I created a program to help people take a quantum leap toward attaining the success that has eluded them in the past. I will share with you the tools that I extracted from years in the trenches helping the most stubborn cases succeed.

Health: Is It Definable?

Many people define "health" as the state of "not being sick." I think "not being sick" is a lousy definition of health!

Dorland's Medical Dictionary defines health as, **"a state of optimal physical, mental and social wellbeing, and not merely the absence of disease and infirmity."**

I like Dorland's definition. It works for me.

Health is a work in progress. Defining health is as challenging and elusive as trying to define a river. I picture the concept of health as having the shape, body, and characteristics of a river. A river is ever changing. It is never the same from moment to moment. Our bodies have so many variables that affect our physical, mental and social well-being. For example, age, stress, personal finances, physical conditioning, diseases, infections, prescriptive medication, work, responsibilities, our diets, our level of macro and micro nutrients, our work conditions, quality of sleep and hydration. The list could be extensive.

I think the key thing to take away is the insight that

all the categories are essential: Physical, Mental, and Social Well-being.

I have worked with many elite level athletes over the years. Most elite athletes enjoy superior health. I can recall a few elite athletes that were not totally "healthy" in all areas. Gerry, 27 years old, was one patient who fit this profile. On one hand, she could claim "she was never sick a day in her life!" At the same time, she was in an abusive marriage filled with anger, hate, resentment, humiliation and shame. She clearly did not fit Dorland's Medical Dictionary definition of health. She booked an exam and consult to determine if changing her diet would add to her health.

I did a complete history and exam. I also checked her with my Nutritional Kinesiology technique, as well as another type of kinesiology testing that works on the emotional connection to illness. Bingo! Her emotional points were particularly active, especially the grief and anger points. I told her my findings, which must have struck a deep chord, because she burst out crying. She couldn't stop sobbing. Now the whole story came out. She told me that she was stuck in a horrible marriage. Her husband was abusive both physically and verbally. The verbal and mental abuse was happening on a daily basis.

She only came in for about a half a dozen sessions.

I gave her a few chiropractic adjustments, and I tweaked her diet a little. She was already on a Paleo diet. She told me her "story" one piece at a time over those few chiropractic sessions.

I encouraged her to get someone to help her with her marriage/relationship issues. I saw her again about a year later, and she told me her marriage ended in a divorce. I felt like she was healthy at this point. Now she had the "mental and social well-being" components in place that are critical to overall health.

If your goal for health is bragging about all the days you are not sick, you are truly limiting yourself. We all need to raise the bar. Shoot for a higher goal. Striving for optimal physical, mental and social well-being are worthy goals.

You can not buy it or own it. We only rent our health. Hopefully it is a long-term lease. It requires regular payments and upkeep. If you neglect your health, it may rapidly erode. It comes down to getting the big picture. Decide what is important to you, then fight for it!

What Did You Feed the Dog?

(How to feel good from the inside out!)

So much of how we feel and heal is determined by what we put in our bodies. The foods we eat can lead to health and vitality, and conversely can lead to chronic illness, allergies, asthma, skin problems, insomnia, low libido, digestive issues, headaches, hormonal imbalance, exacerbation of autoimmune issues and even cause pain and inflammation in our joints.

It amazes me that people have a disconnection between the foods they eat and how their bodies function. My patients come in and report that they have multiple symptoms that are keeping them from enjoying their lives fully.

When I suggest that they need to get their diet right. I often hear, "Do you think food is playing a component?" "My doctor said that the foods I eat have nothing to do with the fact that I have diarrhea 11 times per day!"

When our family dog has terrible skin, poops on the floor, has diarrhea, retreats to her bed and stays curled up in a ball all day, we automatically ask each other ____? What? Take a guess?

You got it. "What did you feed the dog?" or "Did the dog get into the garbage again?"

Why?

Because, what goes in the dog's mouth, has a lot to do with what comes out the other end. Are you with me?

What goes in the dog has a lot to do with the health of the dog.

Why wouldn't that be sound advice for us, too?

We have perfect clarity when it comes to babies. Most people would never put cola or root beer in a baby's bottle. Of course not! How about a shot of whiskey in the baby bottle, or some chewing tobacco between the cheek and gum? How about artificial flavorings, preservatives, food dyes and colors, and maybe a few teaspoons of sugar or salt to top it off? If you saw someone feeding a baby this way, would you approach the parent and say something? Perhaps that is too confrontational. At least we could agree it would be appalling to witness. Wouldn't you expect that such behavior could cause health issues? It may cause swelling and bloating, some diarrhea, poor sleep, digestive issues in general, failure to thrive, rapid heartbeat, moodiness, attention deficit issues, depression, lethargy or hyperactivity; basically a chronically sick baby.

This is where we see the big blind spot. We see it on the dog. We see it on the baby. Why can't we see it in our adult selves?

Every day in my office, I hear people say to me, "I can't believe the foods that I choose could have that much to do with my health and emotional state."

How old does the baby have to be before we feel it's okay to feed the baby junk food? Somewhere along the line it becomes socially acceptable to feed the human body this way. Before the age of six months, one year, or two years, it may be considered a crime. What age does it become "normal," "socially acceptable," and even "healthy"?

Are you chronically tired and getting sick too often? If you are hormonally out of whack, feeling the blues and if your libido is lower than whale turd on the bottom of the ocean, then it is time to clean up your act. *Quantum Paleo* is so effective because, as you lose weight you clean up little health problems associated with getting old. Aging is a very real challenge. To a greater extent than you can imagine, we choose or do not choose how we age.

If you stick with *Quantum Paleo* for 21 days, you will begin to lose weight and feel fantastic. Your emotional state will begin to balance.

The best test is to commit to a 21-day trial. What if

you were the success story at the back of the book? How would that change your life? When you create your own success story, e-mail it to me. I want to know about it!

Challenge #1

Here is your first challenge. Take out your journal or notebook and **write down your success story before you start the *Quantum Paleo* program!** I'm serious, make it up. Invent it. Crazy idea? Not really.

What if you wrote down everything you want to change as if it already happened?

Here is an example of what it would look like. This is an actual journal entry from a patient that tried this exercise before she attempted the *Quantum Paleo* program. Everything in this "prediction" came true except that she lost 13.2 pounds in 21 days rather than the 11.5 pounds she predicted before she started!

Here is the journal entry.

"Dear Dr. Doug,

Not only did I lose 11.5 pounds in 21 days, but my body never felt better. I am pooping every day like clockwork. I feel recharged in the mornings after a good nights sleep. I am exercising with purpose. My cholesterol and triglycerides are down into a normal range. My Hemoglobin A1c is now normal, too. Did I mention my sex life? Oh boy, has that changed too! My libido is better than it has been in 15 years. In the last few days I started dreaming and planning my future. I want to go back to school and finish my certification so that I can earn more money. I am playing the guitar again. I have so many plans and projects and goals swimming in my head. People at work are noticing, too. They want to know my "secret." One of the biggest shifts was patching things up with my dad. I was certain he would shoot me down when I approached him. It was nothing like I expected. To make a long story short, we are back together. We have some work to do. The funny thing is I find myself with better willpower when I'm not at war with people in my life. Is that possible? I am going to take two days off and then start another round. Next goal: Looking great in a bathing suit for the summer. Thanks Dr. D!"

Write down your results before they happen. Write down exactly how you want your future to unfold. It takes imagination. It may feel ridiculous. Try it. Have the courage. What do you have to lose?

Challenge #2

Okay. That's the body. What about the mind?

I want you to bring back that old hobby that you haven't done in years. It may be knitting, horseback riding, singing in the shower, or playing that old guitar you haven't touched in years. How about photography, watercolors, or finger painting? How about something outdoors like hiking, frisbee, or a fun game of tennis? Begin an activity or a hobby again. It will function as a message to yourself that you are worth it!

Before I created the *Quantum Paleo* program, I used to supervise a 21-day cleanse/detox diet with my patients either in person or over the phone. I've been doing it for over 14 years. This is what eventually became the workshop/support group I taught every Tuesday night in New York City for three years. It was first called the "Eliminate the 3 Whites Diet," then it changed to the "Purification Diet," and then I named it "The Big Sweep."

I always worked in rounds of 21 days. The main difference between the *Purification Diet* and the *Quantum Paleo* program was that I gave my patients herbal supplements that would safely cleanse and detoxify their bodies. It was a very popular workshop. I eventually stopped to be home with my kids more. Everyone lost weight, erased symptoms and watched their health soar. My guidelines were to follow the diet and to try something creative or fun that would bring you joy. My favorite part of the evening was when the participants would share the hobbies and creative pursuits that they reinstated in their lives.

One woman in the cleanse group, Clarice, was caring for her terminally ill husband. They were retired and could not afford a home nurse. She did everything for her husband 24 hours per day for close to a year. She was consumed with taking care of him and never made time to do anything fun for herself. She diligently followed the diet program but "she had no time" to experiment with my suggestions to incorporate a hobby or something creative. She couldn't remember the last time she even smiled, let alone had fun.

One night, she shared with the group that years ago she liked to memorize poems and occasionally recite them to her friends. This was something that in the past made her happy. We all encouraged her to bring a poem into class the following week. She agreed to memorize a poem and recite it to us. The next class, she recited a poem by Robert Frost.

"Stopping by Woods on a Snowy Evening"
by Robert Frost.

Whose woods these are I think I know.
His house is in the village, though;
He will not see me stopping here
To watch his woods fill up with snow.

My little horse must think it queer
To stop without a farmhouse near
Between the woods and frozen lake
The darkest evening of the year.

He gives his harness bells a shake
To ask if there is some mistake.
The only other sounds the sweep
Of easy wind and downy flake.

The woods are lovely, dark, and deep,
But I have promises to keep,
And miles to go before I sleep,
And miles to go before I sleep.

She spoke with such passion, totally transported. I felt goose bumps immediately and was transfixed with her eyes as they started to tear up halfway through the passage.

Thirty-two of us were all sniffling and teary. Not

from the poem as much as from the miracle of transformation that we were witnessing. When she finished, we were absolutely quiet for about 30 seconds, after which we all jumped up to give her hugs and feedback.

It was amazing that she picked that poem. For me the last stanza is about responsibility. I love this poem. Of course, you may see it different from me. The poem always made me aware of the juxtaposition between taking a pause in life to appreciate something simple and special, and the constant pull to get back to our "work" and carry through with our obligations.

Her hard, wooden, emotionless face softened that night. We saw her transform in front of our eyes. We transformed with her.

Remember, health is not merely the absence of disease. It is a balance of physical, mental and social well-being.

To feel good, you need to look on the inside. You will only scratch the surface if your goal is to start and finish the 21 day *Quantum Paleo* program.

Branch out and look for ways that you could install some fun back into your life. Restart a hobby or start a project that will bring you joy.

If you made it this far in the book, then you probably had a thought or an idea pop into your head when I wrote about a creative pursuit or hobby. This is the element of fun or creativity that is sitting in some lonesome corner of your past.

Here's your chance to dust it off and bring it back into your life. Go onto my website and share with me in the Success Stories section what activity you are bringing back into your life. Sharing can inspire and act as a catalyst of transformation for someone else. Don't be stingy. Passively reading this book is not nearly as powerful as actively participating.

In the Success Stories section of my PaleoSoul.com blog, let other readers know what you are committed to bringing back in your life that makes you happy.

The Man in the Arena

Excerpt from the speech "Citizenship In A Republic", delivered by Theodore Roosevelt at the Sorbonne, in Paris, France, on 23 April 1910

"It is not the critic who counts; not the man who points out how the strong man stumbles, or where the doer of deeds could have done them better. **The credit belongs to the man who is actually in the arena**, whose face is marred by dust and sweat and blood; who strives valiantly; who errs, who comes short again and again, because there is no effort without error and shortcoming; but who does actually strive to do the deeds; who knows great enthusiasms, the great devotions; who spends himself in a worthy cause; who at the best knows in the end the triumph of high achievement, and who at the worst, if he fails, at least fails while daring greatly, so that his place shall never be with those cold and timid souls who neither know victory nor defeat."

This may be my all-time favorite quote. The "credit belongs to the person" that participates, that takes on the challenge and fights for something worth fighting for! You must try and try again, regardless of the outcome. Either way, you will never be with those "cold and timid souls who know neither victory nor defeat".

My personal challenge is to stay in the "arena". I have failed at so many things. I have failed at managing my finances, my career, my health and body weight. That is what the *Quantum Paleo* program is all about. The program is a way of life. I should have called it the "Fight For The Life You Want Diet", but it was not as catchy.

Notice Teddy Roosevelt did not say, "The credit belongs to the person who does it perfectly" or "The credit belongs to the person that has a great track record, or has no regrets!" No, he didn't say that. He said, we need to be "in the arena".

Here is how "to do" the diet. You jump in the arena and start. Follow the plan. Be forewarned, that there is always an opponent. The opponent is your temptations, your fears, your self-esteem, your confidence and your critics. This opponent wants to hold you down and make you submit and quit. There comes a time to fight. There is the part of you that wants to quit when it gets tough. You may not lose as much weight as you want the first week, or the second week. You may find yourself constipated or gassy. Just do the 21-Day program anyway. Don't wait for perfection, because it is not coming. Don't wait for the perfect timing on the calendar to start. Do not worry if everything is not perfect. Get in the arena and do your best. That is all I'm asking. It will work, if you do!

Live Out Loud

"I came to live out loud!"
Emile Zola

One of the reasons diets don't work is because people have an escape plan before they start a program. When a person keeps their goals a secret, it becomes easy to abort the mission and return to base. They buy a round trip ticket. Preplanning to return to their normal, comfortable rut, as soon as they venture out away from home.

Tell other people about your plans to transform your health and lose weight. This is what I call "living out loud." It becomes a one-way ticket. You are essentially saying, "When I go over that bridge I am not coming back!"

It's a big difference from the way most people do it. Most people secretly skim the diet book in the bookstore without even buying it. Then they binge over the weekend and Monday morning they begin the diet. They quit by Wednesday. It was so secretive and sneaky, not even their own spouse knew they were on a diet. They may even say to their spouse,

"No bread today, I feel too stuffed from the weekend."
Vague isn't it? We are not sure if they have started
anything. Worst of all is that this same person doesn't
know if they have started something either. This is
an example of someone dabbling with the diet. They
will most likely quit within a few days. The voyage is
doomed before it leaves the harbor!

Imagine going into battle with this person?

"I got your back for a few seconds. When things get
tough, I'm outta here!"

Challenge #3

Decide to "live out loud"!

Declare that you are doing the *Quantum Paleo* program. Tell at least five people other than your significant other. Share your goals with people that are
important in your life.

Congratulations! You just increased your chances of
success by 95%.

The Gateway to Success

To enter the Kingdom of Success, you must first pass through a gateway. Blocking your path is the biggest badass opponent of all. The opponent you must face is <u>yourself</u>! This next challenge is critical. It is the step that most people skip. Think of this step as a ritual or a ceremony.

You are about to enter the *Quantum Paleo* arena and climb into the "Octagon". It is time to fight for your life and reclaim your health and body! You are cloaked with a cape of failure as you approach the fighting cage. The cape needs to be dropped. The cape represents your fears, regrets, self hate and past failures.

Yes, you can skip ahead and approach this diet mechanically. Let me ask you this question? Why aren't you at your ideal weight right now? Why did you buy this diet book? I know you have <u>not</u> mastered your weight, or health, or you would not be reading this book. Are you like me and have been on a roller coaster of gaining and losing weight your entire adult life? Have you been heavy as long as you can remember? Have you tried other programs before, only to revert to your original spot or worse?

I'm going to show you how to save time. If you complete this challenge, you will find it easier to reach and maintain your ideal body weight. The diet is explained in "Round 7." It's not rocket science. It is four to five meals per day, with an optional snack if you need it. The diet consists of proteins, vegetables, nuts and seeds, some fruit, lots of healthy fats, little starch and zero dairy and sugar! Drink lots of water and exercise consistently and frequently.

That is it. Grains and legumes are not on the diet?

Not much, huh?

Were you expecting some gimmicks? Is it better when there is some weird element to set the diet apart? How about a diet where you have to suck on a lemon before every meal? How about a diet where you have no fat and only one solid food meal a day? How about a diet where you take enough herbal laxatives to poop out your spleen on the sidewalk?

Well that is not happening here. My *Quantum Paleo* program is about making a mental shift. If you have a shift, it becomes exponentially easier to lose weight. When you shift your mind you can accomplish anything with your body, health and almost any aspect of your life that you choose. Today there are many clever diets in the bookstores. The wisdom in *Quantum Paleo* is so simple you may miss it.

The word "diet" has a Greek derivation, and it means "Way of Living".

During the first 21 days of the diet, you will tighten down on the foods you consume. You will eat clean. You will eat on intervals. You will eat smaller portions. There is nothing weird, or bizarre that you have to do. Otherwise, you will be setting yourself up for something you can not maintain. I'm going to ask you to have an entire day of eating healthy. Then the next day, do it again. Now repeat this discipline for 21 days in a row. There are no gimmicks. When the 21 days are over, decide if you need to do another round? If you need to continue, take three days off and start again. If you are truly happy with your body after one round, then proceed to the section of this book called "Round 8" and read "Staying In The Pocket."

Quantum Paleo breaks down like this:

Preparation

   A) Deciding: What you are fighting for?

   B) Get your mind right.

Taking Action

   A) Doing the program.

   B) Perform one or more Rounds (21-day units).

Staying in the pocket

A) Stay on Top!

B) How to maintain and improve.

Stay Connected

A) Plug into my blog or other blogs that inspire and inform you.

B) Continue to educate yourself on health.

C) Join a community of people that stay fit.

Question

Are you going to be like I was in India and watch from the sidelines? This translates to buying this book, or reading it in the snack area of Barnes and Noble for an hour, then leaving it for someone else to put away because you decided the book is not for you.

Quit now! That is what my instructor said to me. Quit now! Or, get in there and play as if your life depends on it.

I'm telling you right now *Quantum Paleo* is not the best diet ever written. There is always something that everyone thinks is better. "The grass is always greener …" This program works. It works because it is accessible and it gets to the core of how and why we change. It will work for you, too.

When you fight, or compete, or dance, or make love, there comes a moment when you have to stop

thinking and analyzing and being technical. There comes a time to be in the moment and just do the task at hand.

"Leap and the Net Will Appear!"

This diet works if you do!

Are you ready to drink from the goblet?

Here it is …

Challenge #4

It's time to forgive yourself. Stop hating your past decisions. Let go of your regrets.

Forgiving yourself sets you free:

Free to lose weight.

Free to be happy.

Free to be in love … again.

Free to be healthy.

Free to give your body exactly what it needs.

Free to transform your life.

Yes, you can bury this book in a time capsule and do 10 more years of psychotherapy and then attempt to get your body on track. That is one way.

Here is what I do with patients in my office. Purchase an ordinary notebook or journal.

Write on the top of the page: "A list of all my regrets." Start it off this way.

A list of all my regrets (long list)

1   If I only …

2   If I would've …

3   If I could've …

4   If I finished …

5   If I never started …

For example:

"If I only took better care of my health."

"If I would have tried harder at my job."

"If I could have seen the economy declining sooner and made the proper adjustments."

"If I only finished high school."

"If I never started smoking cigarettes as a teenager."

Make your own list. It may be long. Keep going. Take as long as you need. Put more regrets on the list. Have the mindset of a cancer surgeon. Cancer surgeons know that there is a significant risk if you leave any of the bad stuff inside the body. You must cut it all out. Don't leave any bad cancer tissue in there. Get it all out! Write it down.

Now circle or put a check mark next to the worst ones. The regrets that have ruined your life.

On a new sheet of paper, transfer over the top five items that you circled. The regrets that you consider the worst. This will be a new list of the **Top 5 Regrets**.

At this point, you have a choice of how you will handle the **Top 5 Regrets** list. Both paths will work. Here is the traditional way. Get counseling. Analyze it, talk about it. Work on it for years if necessary. I'm told that this works for some people.

It's not my way. I prefer you <u>do not</u> do it this way.

Why?

I don't advise spending that much time on something that you will never be able to change.

Please understand that your **"A list of all my regrets (long list)"**, and your **"Top 5 Regrets"** list is nothing but ancient history. The list holds no weight today unless you give it power by constantly focusing on it. Let's say you regret that you didn't graduate from college. Because of this regret, you are not making as much money as you could've or would've. What good does it do thinking about it today? Nothing! Does obsessing about your regrets get you a promotion or a college degree? Does running it over and over in your head increase your income? No!

What if your regret was, "you wish you were closer with your mom before she died"? Now she is dead and you can't patch up that relationship. Here's what you could do. You could write a long letter to her and start off by telling her everything that you felt went wrong in your relationship. You get to go first. Tell her how she made you angry. If you felt she let you down, then tell her in the letter. If you felt at times she was a lousy mother, tell her in the letter. You get to start with the bad. Put it all down. Don't hold back. Now tell her everything you love about her and everything you appreciate about her, too. Tell her how you could have been a better son or daughter. This is a time to be generous with your praise, love and compassion. Close the letter with a paragraph on how you will forgive your mother. Follow that with a few sentences where you ask her to forgive you. Even if you feel convinced it was mostly her fault. Ask her to forgive you. Be authentic with your forgiveness. Taking on this task will heal you on a core level. This is the level you need to be healthy in order to launch all of your transformational goals.

Obviously she will not be able to read this letter, but you will!

Any relationship on your "Regrets" list, either dead

or alive, can be improved. If the person on your list is not reachable because they are dead, in prison, or they won't talk to you, then write a letter and keep it for yourself. This will allow <u>you</u> to heal. Make a decision to forgive yourself, too.

If the 'Regret' on your list is financial, there is nothing you can do about it. It sucks. It happened. Your life is passing you by. Go forward.

My wife and I got scammed a couple of years ago. It amounted to practically our entire nest egg. It was a lot. Trust me. It was similar to the Bernie Madoff scam that everyone knows about. Eight years of saving money working six days per week. Gone. The bad guys went to jail. We never recovered our losses. Not only did we lose everything but it devastated our taxes and credit score. How painful is that? How embarrassing? I can't even put into words the pain it caused. This made my "Top 5 Regrets" list. I was in a slump for almost a year over this. Mostly because we kept thinking we could salvage the situation and that the police would get our money back. We didn't recover a penny. It's over. I had to let it go. I refuse to look back. We needed to move on.

If the 'Regret" has to do with health choices, for example, "I wish I took better care of my body, or I wish I started exercising when I was 20 years old, or I wish I never took up smoking," then change it now.

Decide right this moment *what you are fighting for* and start today.

It's over. Let it go. How about from this day forward you improve every relationship that has meaning for you. It's worth it. Did you know that when I get patients to patch up or end their dysfunctional relationships, they heal rapidly? They lose weight, sleep better, get inspired, start to exercise and literally transform their lives. People signed up to lose 10 pounds in three weeks, and were shocked to experience a major personal breakthrough in some other facet of their lives.

Here is an optional closure. My wife and I have done this together. Put your **Top 5 Regrets** list on a small piece of paper. Put it in a fire safe container, like the fireplace. Say good-bye to the regrets. Kiss it. Then light it (remember to kiss it before you light it!). Watch it burn. Then turn your back. Walk away. Never look back.

Back to the Kingdom of Success …

Look on the floor. There lies your cape of fear, regrets and self-loathing.

Step over the cape. Don't let it touch your feet!

Climb into the arena and get ready to Fight!

Now I'm asking you again. *What are you fighting for?*

Challenge #5

The 10 Questions You Must Answer!

Below is a list of 10 questions that I often ask my patients to answer before they embark on a new health journey. It's easy to skim over them, chuckle about how they don't apply to you, and move on. I feel so strongly about these questions. In fact, if you get really clear on these questions, the diet is easy. Do you only want to lose 10 pounds, or do you want to have a breakthrough in multiple areas of your life? I have much bigger goals for you. I want you to lose weight and take a quantum leap forward in many facets of your life. I have witnessed it so often that I now expect it. I want it for you, too. Here they are. Get a pen and paper and write down the answers. Get emotional about it. Daydream. Visualize. Fantasize. The more you can see this list come alive, the more it will become part of your life!

1   *What are you fighting for?*

2   Who are you fighting for? (Children, spouse, parents, etc.)

3   Other than yourself, when you transform your health and body, whose life will be most affected?

4 What do you want to weigh, and what date do you want to set to attain that goal? (Ex. 154 pounds by 11/1/2013)

5 What area of your health or body needs to improve the most?

6 What disease or condition do you think your body is most vulnerable to as you grow older? (i.e. "Cancer runs in my family," "My mother has diabetes," "I worry about heart disease," "I'm afraid if I don't get a handle on my obesity I will die before my time," etc.)

7 What area of your fitness and conditioning do you need to improve most and/or maintain now? (Strength, endurance, flexibility etc.)

8 What are things that you have not been able to do in the recent past? (Walk, run, climb, travel, dance, lift heavy things, etc.)

9 Who would be unhappy if you attained your goals? (This may be someone that you have in your life that wants you to fail)

10 What specific goals would you attempt to accomplish when your health, energy levels and body are at its best? (Career, pay off debt, finance, education, relationships, hobbies, learning a new language, travel, learn an

instrument, write a book, run a marathon, climb a mountain, etc.)

First, write down the questions in a journal or notebook, and then formulate answers for each one. Next re-read the questions and answers, and then journal about how they make you feel. Journal about what memories it brings up. Journal about your dreams. Keep your notebook in a private location. Only show your list to someone if they are showing you their list. No exceptions. Only people that have made their own list will truly be able to support you unconditionally.

Blah, Blah, Blah

I am the king of excuses. How about you?

Excuses, aka: Could've-Would've-Should've!

Here are some examples ...

If my mother/father was only ____. If my spouse was only ____. If I only finished that project. If I only didn't hang out with those people. If I only stuck with that path that I was on.

Listen, I don't hate your excuses. I'm too busy hating my own. Okay ... I hate yours too, because it reminds me of how much I hate my own excuses!

Regrets annihilate life! Regrets are worse than cancer. They fester, they rot your core, they rot your soul and they metastasize. They keep resurfacing like a monster in a horror movie. Regrets travel through your body and eat you alive. They drain out your blood and rob you of your life. (Can you detect that this is an area that I have a strong opinion?)

Here is another example ...

If I only did or didn't _____. What? Come on! You got one, too!

I got mine. I finished in the top twenty of my high school and went to Cornell University and then dropped out after three years. Twelve years later, I finished my college degree. It wasn't an Ivy League one, either. Partied too much. I pissed it away. I really regret that. I left school, moved to New York City and got some occasional work as an actor, then a waiter, bartender and a limo driver. I don't regret moving to NYC and pursuing acting. I regret not finishing up at Cornell University. I feel that one decision set me back about 10 years. I was on a great path, and chose one that made my life very difficult.

I've got other regrets. We all do, but I choose not to watch the reruns.

If I only…

It's possible to reinterpret those moments we regret or even forgive ourselves of those decisions. In my case, I am now choosing to view the decision to leave school as part of my life path. In a way, it was my fate. I am exactly where I should be in this moment. I eventually finished college and chiropractic school, too. All the things I've done have made me arrive here as the person I am today. I'm grateful for my wife and children, and so many things that I wouldn't have today if I went another way.

But you know what?

Blah, Blah, Blah!

Blah, blah, blah is the sound your sad story makes to another person's ears.

I'm not talking about the stories about hope and redemption. We want to hear those stories. Everyone gladly listens to stories about love and triumph. Stories about perseverance under adversity are always welcomed. I love those stories. Can't get enough, actually.

But stories about regret … Blah, Blah, Blah!

Here's a little secret. Nobody wants to listen to your sad list of regrets. Nobody really cares. Nobody. Not your spouse. Not your best friend. Not your mother. Especially not your children. That is why we pay therapists a lot of money to sit still and listen to our regrets. Whenever someone is forced to listen to our sad regrets, the only words they hear are Blah, Blah, Blah! Trust me on this one. Even if I'm wrong, what good does it do? Stop rehashing it because it is costing you too much.

Here is another insight.

Your regrets are keeping you from losing weight!

They are keeping you from getting healthy! They are keeping you from healing your life in every way!

No regrets! Agreed?

Quantum Paleo starts in the next chapter. This is it. The time is here. No one is making you do this. No one can put a piece of cake in your mouth and sabotage your success. Only you can. Are you already planning to fail? Are you formulating your excuses? Or are you planning to win? It's more than a diet. There is a possibility to use this tool, or strategy as a catalyst to change everything in your life.

How could that be?

Answer: This program allows you to choose to be responsible for your life. If you choose to go forward. If you let go of excuses and regrets. Then you can transform your body, your mind and eventually any aspect of your life. You will create momentum.

What if you are old, or young, or have a physical handicap and it takes you twelve rounds of 21 days to get to the level of health that would make you healthy and happy? Just do it!

What if you have no time, money and endless obstacles? Blah, Blah, Blah. Make it work. Or don't!

When I was 22 years old, and living in Los Angeles, I had a friend named Catie. She lived across the street.

One day we were talking about our childhood and I made the mistake of complaining about my parents' divorce. I told her my entire "blah, blah, blah" story. I was convinced that I would be so much further along if I did not have to deal with those obstacles from my past. In other words, I was reciting my regrets list.

It was now her turn.

She told me about the day she found her father dead, hanging from a rope in her house at the age of 12 years old. She told me that her mother committed suicide six months later. Catie and her four siblings were split up among four sets of aunts and uncles in four separate homes. Each family was spread out across the country and the siblings hardly saw each other again the rest of their childhood. Catie is bright, funny and extremely creative. Catie never complained or made excuses. If anyone could get leverage out of their regrets, it was Catie, but she never did. The point is ... everyone has a worse story than you!

We all know people that interact with their Blah, Blah, Blah story as if it was their lifetime achievement. It became their greatest defining moment! Some people persevere against all odds, while others stagnate or decline when bad stuff happens. We all must choose.

I guess what I'm trying to say is that there are a million reasons to fail at *Quantum Paleo*. There are only two or three reasons you won't.

When your write down on an index card: What you are fighting for? You will have all the reasons you need to succeed.

What are you fighting for?

Challenge #6

Write it down, now!

Round 5
Tale of the Tape
The Wish List

When I teach a workshop I often ask a question that I heard another speaker say years ago. I don't know who gets credit for the idea; as long as you know it's not my idea. It is probably Brian Tracy or Jim Rohn.

First, I ask workshop participants to write down their goals. I notice many people often censor and filter their authentic dreams and desires. They may write down, *I want to make 10% more income this year. I want to cut my cigarettes down by three per day.* Or, *I want to drop half a pound per week for the next four weeks.* Translation: I'm playing it safe!

Why?

Adults have been around long enough to be disappointed. We have had our bubble burst more than once.

We have stopped believing in Santa Claus.

Did you ever see a little kid on Santa's lap? The child has zero filters. When Santa asks, "What do you want this Christmas?"

The kid will start thinking big.

"I want a new house, pony, bicycle, flat screen TV and I want to go to Disney. I also want to grow six inches in the next two weeks and …"

Does the kid say, "I want to get a pony, but that's only if my mutual fund performs better than it has in recent years?"

No! He just says what he or she really wants.

Here is the big question. What would you ask for if you were a kid sitting on Santa's lap?

That's what I want to know.

Get out a piece of paper and write down how much weight you want to lose. Write it down.

Who wrote the number? Was it the adult part of yourself or the little kid? I want the kid inside of you to write the goals down because you may be too cautious or tentative.

Do you get the idea that people are afraid to put down anything big? Small is safe. Big is scary.

Give the pen, or crayon, to the child part of you and

let him or her answer these questions.

I asked these same questions in the last section. I am not having a senior moment, by the way! I want you to answer them again. Try to forget the way you answered them before. Get out a fresh page in your journal. This time think big! Let your uncensored mind pick up the crayon or pencil and write down your real goals. Then you can check back and see what you put down before. If you haven't participated up until now, that's okay, pick up the pencil and get started. No regrets!

How much weight do you <u>really</u> want to lose?

How many Rounds of 21 days will it take?

How many times per week will you exercise?

What type of exercise will you do?

What other health goals do you have?

What internal areas of your body need to improve (heart, lungs, immune system)?

When was the last time as an adult you were happy with your weight?

What are you fighting for?

What is the second most important thing you are fighting for?

Who are you fighting for?

Anyone else?

What would change for you if you met your goals?

How would you see yourself differently?

What would others think about your progress?

When was the last time you really lived your life full out?

Do you plan on doing *Quantum Paleo* with a partner?

Do not skip this step or I will come to your house and hand you a crayon and do it with you!

The late motivational speaker Jim Rohn said, *"The future does not get better by hope, it gets better by plan. And to plan for the future we need goals."*

And this one by W. W. Ziege:

"Nothing can stop the 'person' with the right mental attitude from achieving his goal; nothing on earth can help the 'person' with the wrong mental attitude." W.W. Ziege

Make your wish list now! It is not a request.

The Only Diet That Counts

You must measure. We need to know our starting point. We need to know how much we weigh. We need to know our waist measurement. Our chest measurement. Our hip measurement.

Buy a tape measure and measure around your belly button. Do it three times and get the average. Write it down. Do not have your clothing in the way.

Next measure your chest three times across the nipples. Arms relaxed and down. Write down the average.

Next measure your hips. Measure around the largest part of your buttocks.

Can you get someone to measure your % body fat? Write it down and date it (This is informative if you can get it, but it is not necessary to proceed).

Here are other things you can measure. They are optional. It is always fun to see all the things that change once you apply yourself.

If you decide to order blood work, please make sure you do the following lab tests.

Make sure they include a lipid profile.

Hemoglobin A1c (this is a great test to see how your blood sugar has averaged over the last three months).

Cholesterol

Triglycerides

LDL

HDL

Morning Glucose

Request the whole panel with the Hemoglobin A1c added to the package.

Daily Caloric Intake

Go to my website http://PaleoSoul.com and find my "Tools" page. Plug your numbers into the Daily Caloric Intake calculator and learn examples of your daily caloric intake requirements.

Then divide that number by five. That will be the average of how many calories you will have per meal. Please notice that you can change the amount of exercise you average per week. You may run the calculations for three workouts per week, and then again for five workouts per week.

For example, let's say that your calculations show 2000 calories per day. Divided by five meals, equals 400 calories per meal.

Three scrambled eggs with mushrooms and ¼ avocado, in an omelet with a double espresso totals just under 400 calories.

If you are a smaller person, it will be scaled down. For example, if the calculator suggests 1200 calories (petite person) that will comprise of three meals of 300 calories each and two snack meals of 150 calories each.

I really want you to use the Daily Caloric Intake Calculator as a starting place.

Next step is to track your calories for the first 21 days. At the very least track your calories for the first week. This will teach you where you stand. Many mobile phones have calorie tracker apps. You can also go to livestrong.com or sparklepeople.com and use their database and calorie trackers for free. Most of my patients use, My Fitness Pal, http://www.myfitnesspal.com. Keep in mind that these sites do not teach Paleo eating.

Counting and measuring is tedious but it works. Remember, it is not for the rest of your life. I want you to count your calories for at least seven days, but preferably all twenty-one days of your first round. If you are someone that needs to lose a lot of weight, than I suggest you stick with your daily input of calories on My Fitness Pal or something similar for six to twelve months or until you have reached your goal.

Once you know your numbers we can always make modifications. For example, if you are not on track to lose weight after five days, we may need to trim another 100–150 calories per day from the daily caloric intake.

Are you exercising four to five times per week?

Are you sleeping as well as you possibly can?

Are you drinking your water consistently?

In order to master your body and maximize results, you must write everything down.

If you had a coach, he or she would be writing it down for you. Be your own coach and write it down.

Knowing your math and collecting data will safeguard you from failing.

The first 21 days I recommend using a five-meals-per-day plan with an optional snack if needed. A few "Paleo" lifestyle experts recommend less meals per day than the five that I recommend. In my clinical experience, I see better results when the patient starts with an average of five feedings or meals per day. I want to keep morale high. After one or two cycles of 21 days, I may transition my patient over to four meals per day.

A Few More Things You Can Do.

Keep a journal.

I always keep a journal. I have been keeping a journal since I was 18 years old. I constantly write down my thoughts, my goals, my plans and my dreams. I don't always write every day. However, year after year I fill up my journals and start new ones. My goals are so lofty that they border on delusional and probably would appear that way if my journal "fell into enemy hands." I don't share my journal with anyone. It's my stuff.

Keeping a journal will help you stay on track. You can write down your measurements and your goals for safe keeping.

Start a blog.

Have you ever thought of blogging? Here is your chance to blog about your experience and journey of getting into the best shape of your life. I promise it will keep you on track. The moment you declare your goals to the public, it will intensify your commitment. This is a way that you can "live out loud". You can even start a blog for free through Google at http://blogger.com.

Take before and after pictures.

Take a simple photograph in short pants or a bathing suit with your arms by your side. Then take a side view and a view of your back. It is powerful to see your before and after pictures after meeting your goals. Most cell phone cameras will be sufficient to accomplish this task.

Here is another challenge:

Document your success story.

I want success stories for a future book. Can you write a short essay on your experience and results and then send me the report via e-mail? What was your starting point? How long did it take you? What were your results? What were you fighting for? How did it feel? What happened in other areas of your life; relationships, finance, career, creativity, health, etc. The essay should be no longer than 500–700 words. Send me your before and after pictures if you have them. Let me know if I can use it on my blog site, or even my next book. Also, let me know how you want your name to appear. Some people want their first name and last initial to be recorded. When people choose to "live out loud" with their goals, they create an invincible wave of momentum.

To Weigh or Not To Weigh …

That is the question!

Not for me. I am a huge proponent on weighing yourself every day.

During the *Quantum Paleo* program, I want you to weigh yourself every morning for 21 days. First thing when you get up. Use the toilet. Get naked. Then get on the scale.

Why?

We need to know. The initial phase of this diet is only 21 days.

There are many good reasons to weigh yourself every day for the first Round of 21 days.

I don't want to lose an entire week wondering if you are on track. If you are not progressing after a few days, you need to re-evaluate your math (calories) and your exercise frequency and intensity. Being in the dark about your status is not acceptable.

Most diet plans recommend that you weigh yourself once per week. Once per week is considered sound advice because it may be upsetting to see your weight fluctuate throughout the week. I am not negotiable on this topic. Weigh yourself every day. That is your homework. I want you to know what your weight is every day.

There is power in knowing.

For example:

I want you to know if you hold onto water on Days 10–14 of your menstrual calendar.

I want you to know how much your weight swings when you hold water before, during and after your period. I also want you to write it down and put it in a journal.

I want you to learn the exact day of the month you can expect a weight shift. Are you more water-retentive during ovulation (mid-month) or are you holding more weight before, during or after your menstruation?

I want you to know if you are holding on to water if you eat too much sodium.

I want you to know how much the scale jumps when you cheat and have four glasses of wine and a peanut butter and jelly sandwich at midnight.

I also want you to know how much a strict diet and a great session of cardio can help you to stay on track. I want you to know what four cardio sessions per week can do for your "numbers" compared to two or three.

Weighing yourself everyday holds you accountable.

If you have a deadline, then you need to measure. Twenty-one days! Make every day count.

Why do I have my clients weigh themselves every day?

I know this is against the popular info. I'm coming from a different point of view, so hear me out.

A big part of what I teach is for people to be on the path to master their bodies. Can we master our bodies? I certainly haven't mastered mine. I am trying to learn about my body every day. That is the path to building health. I ask patients to weigh themselves every day for several months if they need to lose a lot of weight.

For example, a patient comes into my office and wants to lose 75 pounds. I learn that this person has not exercised in years. I need them to take a daily inventory. I do not want them to just "shut up and do what I tell them". I want them to be a partner with me in losing weight.

The most important goal is for them to become responsible in building their own health. I want them to weigh themselves every day for the initial 21 days. I want them to count calories for the first three weeks. I want them to look at their poop, track their sleep and their water, too. As people do this, they start to learn how their body functions. Keeping track of this data, measuring and observing, they will learn that all the big mysteries of weight fluctuation are predictable. Once they understand that they are responsible for their own body, they are on the road to mastery.

I find when patients learn to "know their bodies" they have the ability to control their weight and to some extent their health.

How often do we hear, *"I don't know what happened... I somehow gained 30 pounds in the last two years"*?

If you are not seeing the scale move in a downward trend, then you need to eat less and/or exercise more. If you still do not see results, you may want to work closely with your doctor. It may be necessary to determine if you have a metabolic or hormonal reason that is keeping your body from losing the weight.

Know your numbers. It's powerful!

Counting Calories?

I hate counting calories. I don't recommend it.

Actually, sometimes I do!

When?

I got ahead of myself. Let me back up. When it comes to diet coaching, I have typically three types of clients.

Client 1: 25–45 years old, in decent or good shape but has 10–15 pounds to lose. They were athletic throughout their lives and probably are exercising on a semi-regular basis. This type of person needs some education on food choices and will do very well with adopting a "Paleo" way of eating. They don't need to weigh themselves every day, they probably don't need to count calories. They need to simply eat well on a consistent basis and be consistent with their workouts, too. Over a few months they will shift into their ideal body composition.

Client 2: Any age, needs to lose a lot of weight. They have let themselves go for a long time. They may not remember a time when they were ever in good shape. They are not athletic and/or haven't been for years.

This type of person I encourage to weigh themselves every morning for 21 days. I also have them count calories for at least seven days. Twenty-one days is preferable.

Client 3: Has had a huge health scare. They need to turn around their way of eating because their life and health depend upon it. I've had a lot of these patients over the years. I often have them do my 21 day Paleo Purification Program, which is basically my *Quantum Paleo* diet with a 21 day herbal detox kit added in. When the detox/cleanse is finished, I have them follow my *Quantum Paleo* program as a lifestyle regimen. This person we advise to weigh and calorie count on a daily basis for the first 21 days. This type of client needs to do the program 100%. No compromising on the program. Zero grains. Zero legumes. Zero sugar. Zero alcohol. Zero Dairy. Their life and health depend on it.

Here's the reasoning …

Clients #2 and #3 need to weigh themselves every day and count calories because they don't have the "innate" monitor that many athletes and super healthy people rely on. Putting them on the perfect "Paleolithic" type of diet is not enough.

They need to start to get to know their bodies better.

I recommend that my patients start to eat healthy

proteins, veggies, fruits, seeds, nuts and good healthy fats. I want them to drink water as their main beverage. This is the *Quantum Paleo* plan.

I also want them to weigh themselves every morning for 21 days. This is against most weight loss programs. Weight Watchers, for example, recommends that you weigh yourself once per week.

I want my patients to get to know their bodies. I want them to journal how they react to food, sleep and even look at their bowel movements every day, too.

I want them to count calories for a minimum of seven days, twenty-one preferably, and maybe as long as six months to a year.

I want the client/patient to become responsible for their body. Some people have no clue why their bodies gain or lose weight.

Weigh yourself daily. Count what goes in and what comes out. People often forget that they will gain weight when they consume more calories than they burn. A person loses weight when they consume less calories then they need for maintenance. It's important to know the "math" of your body.

Think of an attentive, observant mother of a newborn baby. She looks at the poop. She listens to the burps. She looks at the skin. She smells the baby. She washes the baby. She observes and reacts. The mother really gets to know the baby because she is responsible for the child's wellbeing.

If the poop is looking funky, that may indicate a potential health issue. Time to make an adjustment to the diet. If it does not resolve it may be time to seek an appointment with a healthcare provider. Who is taking care of your body today? Many adults have not paid attention to their bodies in decades.

I get e-mails from experienced "Paleo" people that argue that calorie counting is not necessary for them.

If you are an athlete or a nutrition savvy person, you already know this stuff. You can skip over this advice. Remember, I see people in my practice that are not as advanced as you. I meet people in my practice that need a lot of help.

Making a quantum shift is more important than simply losing weight. People need to have a shift in their whole relationship to food and their health.

Know your "math" and learn to make changes that support your health and body composition.

Round 6
The Pre-Fight

Sex and Wine

I decided to allow two glasses of wine per week on *Quantum Paleo*, but sex is unlimited.

Why?

Sex for some people is the only time they are not thinking about food.

When I was attending chiropractic school I had a nutrition professor, Dr. T., who was disliked by the majority of students. I actually found Dr. T. inspiring. When it came to the way people should eat, he was strict. He was a perfectionist. Unbendable.

Outside of teaching, he had a private practice in Atlanta, Georgia. He consulted with patients that were extremely ill. Utilizing only diet and nutrition, he was able to turn around many long-term chronic situations.

My wife Rachel and I decided to take Rachel's mother, Trudy, to see Dr. T. Trudy was in decent health overall, but already in her late 70's she was experiencing chronic arthritis pain in her knees, shoulders and spine. She also had a recurring upper respiratory infection every winter.

Dr. T. ordered several tests, including a food allergy test (Elisa IgG Food Assay). I still order this test for my patients in my office. After reviewing the results, he told Trudy to eliminate all grains, dairy and sugar, as well as another dozen minor foods that showed up on her blood test.

Trudy was a World War II concentration camp survivor. She had been brutalized, imprisoned, starved and separated from her brother and mother who were eventually executed at another camp.

Somehow she survived those years. She told us that during her incarceration she would dream about the chance to eat a simple piece of bread and creamy chunk of brie. After the war, she relished eating a baguette with a slice of brie every afternoon.

Now, Dr. T. was demanding that she quit her bread and cheese.

Trudy didn't want to see Dr. T. in the first place. Rachel and I strong-armed her into the original appointment. Trudy lasted about three minutes on that diet! She didn't give a crap about following his advice.

Here's my point.

When I sit down with a patient, I ask them about their health and body goals. I try to find out, *What they are fighting for?* I then suggest little incremental steps. Reachable. Attainable.

I find out what they currently eat and try to set up a customized program that is as close as possible to the foods that they already eat and enjoy. If a patient has lived their life mostly eating pizza, junk food and low quality foods in general, I will ask them to start eating healthier meats and animal proteins. Next I try to have them add some vegetables to their diet. I want them to switch from sodas and fruit juices to drinking water as their main beverage. Eating good quality ingredients is a priority.

The 21-day diet is a fast blast. I will ask you to eliminate a few of your favorite foods.

In Round 8 of this book, you will learn to live with certain trade-offs. A trade-off is when you get to keep this in your life, if you can give up that. Another example is with exercise. Some people choose to exercise more so they can maintain their ideal body weight. This allows them to eat some fun foods occasionally. After reaching your ideal weight with *Quantum Paleo*, you can treat yourself to a glass or two of wine while dining at a restaurant. For example, order a steak with a salad, a side dish of veggies, but be committed to avoiding the bread and dessert. This is the trade off; have the wine but skip the bread and dessert. This is the way you can maintain your hard won results. Do you want to continue to look good naked? Or what?

If Trudy was my patient, I would have kept her on the bread and brie!

Why?

A few reasons.

If I did a proper interview, I would have discovered that eating brie and bread was the high point of her day. She was 77 years old. She was fighting to keep her brie and baguette in her routine until the day she died.

She was thin. She never over ate. She did a swimming workout five mornings a week. She had many good things in place. The only prescription medication she was taking was for Type 2 diabetes.

My plan would have been to allow her to have brie and bread every afternoon. As a starting point! Then plan the rest of her day around it. She needed to eat tiny meals every three hours. I was surprised to learn that she was never advised about her diet and blood sugar maintenance. I would have given her a few supplements to take daily. Her water intake was very low and needed to be corrected. I would have suggested she take out all other dairy, grains and sugar, other than her brie and bread snack.

Why would I keep her on dairy and grains? Am I contradicting myself? No. Remember, I am first a healthcare provider. I am not a "Paleo Evangelist". Trudy never said she was interested in a "Paleo" diet. Ramming "Paleo" down her throat made her quit within 24 hours. Who won? Nobody.

In my experience of working with patients, I have found it is better to listen to the patients and figure out where they are and what level of commitment they have. Then start to ratchet it up from there. If Trudy was educated on the dangers of dairy and grains as it was revealed from her blood test, she would know that the brie and bread were her "cheat" foods. Then, as we eliminated all other grains and dairy, she could then decide how often she wanted to "cheat."

Many of my patients get momentum once they start to feel better. They begin to gain strength and make better choices. They begin to take responsibility for their own health. Trudy may have had great success with being off of grains 95% of the day. We will never know. Trudy ate bread and brie until the day she died in a fatal car accident a few years later. *We love you "Oma".*

I have other patients that are willing to radically change everything within seconds of my suggestions. My job is to provide a path for multiple types of personalities to get well and conquer their health issues.

If Trudy's problem was Inflammatory Bowel disease, or Celiac disease, that would be a different story. The tougher the disease, the more difficult choices will need to be made. If she did have a life-threatening bowel disease directly related to grains, I would have had a very different conversation with her.

Back to the wine.

Twenty-one days is relatively short. I prefer if you can do *Quantum Paleo* with little to no wine. If I designed a plan without wine as an option, 40% of the participants would cheat. 50% of you are fine without wine for 21 days; 10% don't drink, so they have no issue either way.

I decided to build two glasses of wine per week into the plan. I'm also going to teach you how to do it and not get off track.

Two glasses per week! Not three. Not five. Zero is allowed,too!

I feel there is more to learn about yourself, while drinking two glasses per week than zero glasses. Two glasses teaches you moderation. If I bully you into abstinence, it makes you yearn for Day 22. Then the minute *Quantum Paleo* is over, you will want to get hammered.

Enjoy a glass of wine midweek and another on the weekend. Or have both glasses on the same night. Whether your preference is red wine or white, I don't care. No beer or hard liquor, please.

If you are going to have some wine, then tightly monitor your calories that day. Perform an extra session of cardio during the week. You may also trim down your calories a little per meal. Smaller portions. Each glass of wine is approximately 150–190 calories. Can you mathematically work in 150 calories into your daily intake? Can you incorporate 300 calories of wine into your daily total and still be on target? You must think this way.

In other words ... build it in!

Drinking every night doesn't work.

Yes, Dr. T's "perfect diet" is better than my *Quantum Paleo* for sick people. I have put very sick people on Dr. T's "perfect diet" and it yields great results. Only about 1-3% of the population can be "perfect" month after month. One of the goals of my practice has been to get great results with a large percentage of my client base. I want people with weak willpower to get results, too.

After you have achieved your goal weight and desired

level of health, you will move into the Post-Fight program. This is discussed in detail in Round 8 of this book. It will include one small glass of wine at dinner on three nights per week. On a fourth night you can have two glasses of wine. That's four nights per week! First you need to learn the balancing act.

If you are dealing with a major illness, I recommend that you work one-on-one with a nutrition expert. This book will not be comprehensive enough for the person that is in crisis. *Quantum Paleo* is for relatively healthy people that want to take it up a notch, reclaim their vitality and turn back the clock to a time they were happy with their bodies.

My plan is to help you lose weight fast enough without losing hope. I also want to include some comfort foods to keep you happy. I have used this program with my NYC patients over the last 14 years. Every year I cull it down and simplify it. Simple works. Complicated is for scholars and researchers.

Sex.

You can have as much sex on this diet as you want. It is great exercise, you burn calories and it typically improves your outlook on life!

I thought if I titled this section "Sex and Wine" you were more likely to read it.

What you need to take away from this section:

Don't be perfect. I want you to be near-perfect in short bursts of 21 days. Learn to have balance and exercise moderation. If you like wine, or chocolate (dark chocolate is better) then "make it work". It may take cutting down over there, to have some choices over here. It may take making exercise a bigger part of your life.

"Sex and wine" are really metaphors for special moments, treats and indulgences that may show up in our week that will challenge you to stay on track.

Let's make room for those special indulgences and learn to make them work!

Did You Go?

"Did you go?" My Grandma Irma would ask me this when I would stay over her house for the weekend. She was very concerned about my bowel movement and frequency of production. The embarrassing part is that she was still asking me this question when I was 14 years old. Sometimes in front of my friends. And eventually in front of my first girlfriend. I must confess, this probing interview ritual skipped a generation with my mother and now I am the next "Grandma Irma." I ask my patients the same question!

Question: How many times per day <u>should</u> you have a bowel movement?

Answer: Once per day at the very least. Many nutrition experts will preach that one bowel movement <u>per meal</u> is ideal. I will add that the stool should be well-formed. Some people won't look. Take a look. It's important.

Dr. T., my nutrition professor, always said to work on the bowel first. He felt no matter what the disease or ailment, make sure the bowel was working as well as possible. I found that to be sound advice over the years.

I have interviewed many patients who felt it was okay to 'go' every other day, or every third day. Their doctor told them that every few days is normal. It may be common, but it is not acceptable. Remember, your feces is the waste of your body. Get rid of the waste. Take out the "garbage". Don't let it fester. This is one of the key pillars to building health. Don't ignore it. My observation is that if a person has infrequent bowel movements, they will suffer from chronic health issues either in the present time or in the future. *Quantum Paleo* has a lot of fiber(vegetables and fruit), water, good oils and fats. This will be sufficient for some, while others may need to take a supplement or two to help in this department. If you are going to begin *Quantum Paleo*, you should put "going" every day at the top of your list.

You should be drinking plenty of water. I recommend having a high quality fish oil supplement. A good probiotic should be part of your daily regimen, too. As you eliminate flour, dairy and sugar, you will find your bowel starting to improve. We use an herbal formula in my practice that yields great results and is safe and effective. You must poop every day. I'm serious.

Lose Weight Sleeping

Can you lose weight sleeping?

Answer: Yes!

I went away for five days over the December holiday in 2010. Five days stretched to ten because of the blizzard that hit NYC. Our return flight was cancelled, and Delta Airlines couldn't get us on another flight for an additional five days. At first I was stressing because I had patients on my schedule between Christmas and New Years. After I rescheduled all of my appointments, I tried to enjoy my extra days in Florida with my family. In my case, enjoyment can directly translate to eating and sleeping. Oh, and some wine, too!

As you may or may not know, my wife and son are both classically trained chefs. Anywhere we go, food is involved. If food were a religion, we would be zealot observers. So, where is this going?

I consumed enough food and wine during this family reunion to feed a family of four in a developing nation for six months. I assumed I gained five to seven pounds during my trip. There was no scale where we were staying, so I couldn't weigh myself during our visit. I usually weigh myself every day. I worked out once during my 10 day stay in Florida with my cousin Jimmy. I know you are hanging on every word at this point. This is a virtual cliffhanger. So, what happened?

When I got home to blizzard buried Brooklyn (we were living in Brooklyn at that time), my scale showed that I lost one pound!

How did this happen? Maybe I didn't eat as much as I thought. No, I ate an enormous amount. Ask my wife. She observes everything and doesn't miss a thing I indulge in. I ate much more than I normally eat. I also had sweets, cookies and ice cream, almost every day. Boy, I was really off track, wasn't I?

The difference was that I slept a lot.

When I am on my normal work schedule in NYC, I typically go to bed at 11:30pm, and wake up at 4:45 a.m. I would say I averaged 5.5 hours of sleep per night in the past seven years.

For 10 days in Florida, I averaged nine hours per night. Slacker! Sloth! Sooey!

Why is this significant? In one word … Cortisol!

Cortisol: Is a hormone that is made in your adrenal glands and secreted into your bloodstream. The adrenal glands directly or indirectly have an effect on almost every cell in your body. The adrenals are the "stress gland" of the body, secreting hormones like epinephrine (adrenaline), cortisol, aldosterone and norepinephrine. The body's physiological response to stress and its ability to react and adapt to that stress is largely the job of the adrenals. Any gland that overworks will eventually under function.

When we are under stress, especially chronic stress, our body releases more cortisol, at higher levels and with increased frequency. This high level will make the body retain fat around the trunk of the body. Hips, abdomen, thighs, buttocks, face, neck and back are the places we gain weight when our cortisol gets high. High cortisol levels disturb sleep and buries you deeper in this vicious cycle. Not only will you experience weight gain, but it becomes an uphill battle to lose weight. In addition, the immune system can get depressed. Blood sugar gets elevated and a decrease in insulin sensitivity can result. Memory, energy levels and your sex drive go downhill, too.

How much sleep is enough? If you didn't use an alarm clock for three to five days in a row and you didn't force yourself to go back to sleep, how much sleep would your body really need? What amount of sleep would be optimal? It's hard to figure out. Many people rely on some form of sleeping pills. Pharmaceutical or "natural" sleep products will both manipulate ones body chemistry. I would be willing to bet that if you could get a minimum of 7.5–8.5 hours of sleep, your health would change and you would have a much easier time with weight loss.

If you have been getting by on five to seven hours of sleep for years and feel great, then you may be the exception. This would mean that you have vibrant energy all day long and get sick less than once per year. If you are sleeping 5-7 hours and have chronic colds, weight you can't lose, having trouble going to sleep and staying asleep, then there is a good chance you have cortisol issues that need to be addressed. The first thing to do is simply get more sleep and see if you get the expected results. If you feel you are "stuck", then it's good to know that cortisol levels can be tested.

Addressing the endocrine system (ie. adrenals, thyroid, hormonal balance and anterior pituitary) from a natural perspective would require a phone or in-person consult. For adrenal issues, chronic fatigue, adrenal fatigue, sluggish thyroid, and hormonal issues, there are safe supplements that I use in my office that are inexpensive and really work. E-mail me if you need info on setting up a phone consult DrDoug@thehealthfixer.com

A good night's sleep changes everything. Inflammation, allergies, memory and libido will improve with improved sleep. Make it your goal to sleep more on a consistent basis. An extra 30–60 minutes of extra sleep will make it significantly easier to lose weight.

Here are some tips:

Your first job is to make sure your room is pitch black. Work on getting your room like a cave. Cover up all lights, alarm clocks, computer monitors and night-lights. Move your alarm clock away from the bed. Get the temperature as close to ideal as possible. For some people that is a little cold, for others it is a little warm. Determine for yourself what temperature helps you stay asleep the longest.

Try to get into a routine. Go to bed as close to the same time every night.

Do not sleep with the television on. Closed eyelids are not enough to block out the light. The porphyrin proteins that make up your red blood cells are sensitive to light and carry this information of light exposure to the brain. This will block the release of the hormone/neurotransmitter melatonin from being released from the anterior pituitary. In short, you won't sleep as well and you will mess up your cortisol balance.

No caffeine after 3:00 p.m. Have a bite of protein at bedtime. Even two ounces of protein at bedtime will help keep your blood sugar balanced.

Sleep is one of the basic pillars of health as far as I'm concerned. Directly behind food, air and water! The question you need to ask yourself is, *are you tired all the time?* Of course, that can come from a number of reasons, but the most obvious place to start is your sleep.

Before you change your room with the suggestions I recommended above, you may want to try this experiment. Keep a record for five days of the time you go to bed, the time you wake up and rate the quality of sleep on a scale of 1–10. Also, take an average of the hours slept over the first five nights.

Then for the next five days, make all of the improvements on your sleep room. Black out the room, get rid of any electrical equipment and adjust the temperature so it is not too warm or cold. Now get to bed earlier. Record all of the new numbers and then compare the data.

Improving the quality of sleep will sharpen your mental acuity, heighten libido, strengthen your immune system and make it easier to manage your body weight. Give it a try.

Exercise or Die!

Pretty strong statement?

It holds a lot of truth.

Maybe a more palatable statement would be, exercise if you want to choose how you die. How about … exercise can change the way you die. As my daughter might say, "I'm being a little dramatic!"

Maybe we can settle on, exercise can change the way we live! Yes, that is much better.

I really enjoyed the book *The Paleo Solution*, by Robb Wolf. He is a research biochemist, athlete, coach, and wrote a great book on the "Paleolithic Diet". He is one of the world's leading experts in Paleolithic nutrition. He writes and lectures about diet, exercise, hormone balance and how we genetically resemble our hunter and gatherer ancestors during the Paleolithic era. He outlines how we should eat to get as close as possible to our genetic potential in weight, health and fitness. Chapter nine was all about the importance of exercise, as it relates to genetic expression. Don't let the subject of genetic expression scare you off. He has a style of making dense material light, funny and informative.

He writes on page 146, *"Our hunter-gatherer ancestors lived an active vigorous life. They and their prehuman ancestors had to expend remarkable amounts of energy to provide food, clothing and shelter. Over the course of millions of years, our genetics were forged with a level of activity not dissimilar from that of an Olympic caliber athlete. This is what our genetics are expecting when we are born into the world. We are literally "born to be fit." An unfortunate side effect of technology and affluence is the physical activity that made our ancestors strong and healthy is all but missing from our sedentary existences. On a molecular level this lack of exercise literally changes who we are."*

Let me give you a quick summary on his main points on genetics. Genotype is the gene pool that you get from your mom and dad. For example, let's say that you have two parents that are elite level athletes and you wind up getting some of their best gene stuff. You have the genetic potential to be an amazing athlete. It is possible for you to do nothing with it, too. A sedentary life can "turn off" that switch.

It still needs to be developed and expressed. That's your phenotype. *"How genes experience the world (be it food, sleep, community, or exercise) influences how these genes are turned on or off and this determines your phenotype,"* writes Wolf.

The image that comes to my mind is the dimmer

switch you have in your dining room. (Assuming you have a dining room. Many of us in NYC have our dining rooms as an extra bedroom!) We can have our genetic dimmer switch operating at full blast if we eat, exercise, sleep and socialize to maximize our genetic potential. Conversely, we can dim down our dimmer switches and operate on a drastically diminished potential. How is that for alliteration!

Let's say you have done very little exercise in the past year. A scientist can take a microarray analysis of your genes/DNA during this "lazy, sedentary state" you've been living in and map out your potential disease profile. This means that they can closely predict what diseases you will succumb to in the next few decades if you remain on this path and don't die of an accidental death.

Here is the good news. Let's say that you got your act together, turned over that new leaf and got in great shape over the next 6–12 months. You got into what I call the "Pocket," lost the excess weight, got on a healthy eating regimen and started to eat a diet that supported your health at a very high level. In other words, you started to eat the way you were designed to eat.

Now if the same scientist did an analysis on your genes at this time, you would be a totally different "you." You would have changed your phenotype. The list of potential diseases would not even resemble the "sedentary" you. It would look like a completely different person!

So, exercise matters. Period.

I hear my patients say, "I don't have enough time to exercise." Or, "I don't like to exercise."

What I'm learning is that it's mandatory. You don't have to like it. It's on the same par as food and air. Imagine if you said, "I don't have time for air!" or "I don't enjoy breathing."

The JAMA, the Journal of American Medical Association, reported that Poor Diet and Inactivity is the second leading cause of preventable death in the USA. This amounts to 16% of deaths that are thought to be preventable. The first is tobacco. The research report estimated the number to be 400,000 people a year die of the result of poor diet and inactivity. That is equivalent to 1000 people a day. Another way to imagine that many people is to contemplate the media outcry if 3 jumbo jets with 300 people each, went down every day for a year. This would be the biggest news story of the century. If people die slowly, because they are misinformed and have been fed disinformation, then that is okay! (Actual Causes Of Death In The United States, 2000. Jama. 2004; 291:1238-1245.)

JAMA concluded the report with the following alarming statement:

"Conclusions: These analyses show that smoking remains the leading cause of mortality. However, poor diet and physical inactivity may soon overtake tobacco as the leading cause of (preventable) death."

On *Quantum Paleo*, I want you to exercise four to five days per week. Remember, phase one is a sprint. Twenty-one days. Fifteen workouts. At least three of the workouts should be 30 minutes or more of an aerobic activity. If you are walking, it should be at a pace that makes you "breathy." If you are more advanced, then try to bring it up a notch. From day one the finish line is in sight. So why hold back?

The cool thing is that you can alter your genetic expression or phenotype, by the choices that you make concerning food and exercise. Your fingers are on your own Rheostat (dimmer switch). So give it a twirl.

Get Fat!

This is a section that could use an entire book to explain it thoroughly. At the back of this book, I recommend a few excellent books that cover it more thoroughly. I really want to stick to my guns and have my book be more focused on the "mind game" and the "what you need to know" rather than the science.

In Robb Wolf's book, *The Paleo Solution,* he covers a very important point concerning cardiovascular disease and saturated fats (Chapter 7, page 109 of the hardcover edition). He said, *"A high intake of saturated fats, in conjunction with a high intake of dietary carbohydrate, is a hell of a combo for an early grave ... If, however, our intake of saturated fat is kept within ancestral limits and we also modify our carbohydrate intake to match that of our ancestors (both in amounts and type), we have little risk of developing CVD (cardiovascular disease)."*

He then sums it up nicely as far as good and bad fats on page 110 of his book.

1. Long chain n-3/ n-6s are good. Fats from grass-fed meats and wild caught fish are good.

2. Ancestral ratios of n-3/n-6 were approximately

1 to 1. Modern ratios are 1 to 10. This is bad.

3. Fats from sources such as corn, soy, safflower, and similar vegetable oils are the source of excessive (n-6) bad fats in our diet. These oils are bad for you.

In other words, there are good fats and bad fats. If we eliminate the horrible processed oils from our diet and the artificial trans fats, like margarine, we will lower our risk of CVD. We need to focus on eating grass-fed meats and wild caught fish, as well as plenty of good oils like olive oil and coconut oil. In addition, avocados and olives are healthy fats. Moderate amounts of fresh seeds and nuts are beneficial, too.

That's it. Keep it simple. If you are interested in the research that supports this, please read Robb Wolf, Loren Cordain, Gary Taubes, Mark Sisson, or Nora T. Gedgaudas's books. They are massively referenced. I also suggest going to the reference section in the back of each book and read some of the sited peer-reviewed research articles on this subject.

How Much Water?

Depends, everyone is different. Most people are not drinking enough. Water in your iced tea, coffee, or artificial beverages does count, but it's an unhealthy way to get it. I had a patient report she never drank water. Zero. When I asked her about this, she corrected herself and said she did have a splash of water with her scotch!

Everyone's needs are different. One widely spread health tip suggests you should drink half your body weight in ounces. Meaning, if you weigh 200 pounds, you would drink 100 ounces of water every day. Others live by the "eight glasses of water per day" golden rule that has been circulating for decades. I have leaned towards advising my patients to drink half their body weight in ounces, because this takes in account the size of the person's body. Variables such as age, weight, activity level, climate/temperature are all factors that need to be considered in determining a proper amount.

The average person is said to obtain 20% of his/her water from foods throughout the day. If the bulk of your diet is vegetables and fruit, this percentage is assuredly higher.

I teach each patient to get to know their body. I really have two categories of patients that I serve. I have healthy athletic people that seem to really know their bodies and they come in for minor issues. They seem to already know how much water, sleep and exercise they need to maintain a balanced healthy life.

The other type of patient that comes to see me is really struggling with building health. They need some guidelines. If that sounds like you, here are some rough guidelines. Start off by drinking a minimum of two liters of water per day for 7 days. After seven days I want you to switch to drinking half your body weight in ounces. Which one works better for you?

When it comes to water, sleep and exercise I feel strongly that we are all biochemically distinct individuals. Water is a category that needs to be adjusted and experimented with on a case by case basis. Be willing to explore on your own. Although your best friend, spouse, personal trainer, massage therapist, chiropractor, or medical doctor may have the perfect amount for you to take; the truth is they really don't know. I do not know, either! Start with a recommended amount, and then "feel" and "experiment" your way to formulating a decision for yourself!

Twenty-one days.

Why?

I used to challenge my patients to do a health-building/weight loss program that lasted 90 days. I even had one that was six months long at one point. It's hard to get people to commit to anything for six months. For example, do you find it difficult to plan your next dental cleaning, six months out? I do.

Twenty-one days is something almost everyone can wrap their brains around. It is hopeful. It is short. It fits on a single page of your monthly planner. You can practically stand on the starting line and see the finish line. It works with people who are intensely driven and it works with people that have difficulty creating inertia.

"Give me 21 days!"

That's what I say.

What if you need more than 21 days to reach your goal?

Don't think about that. Just do the 21 days. Pick a big goal. Mark 21 days on your calendar. Know the exact day you start and the exact day you finish. I should be able to call you on the phone and ask you, "What day are you on?" and you would immediately know that you are on Day 11, or Day 17.

I want you to do at least four work outs per week. Five is better. If you do four, that is 12 workouts in 21 days. Check them off as you do them. It's only 12 workouts. Small bites. How about 15 workouts in 21 days?

"Drop and give me 50 push-ups!"

Can you do it? Most people can't.

Could you do 10 push-ups? Then rest. Now give me another 10. Then give me another ten push-ups, and so on. You could do it if we broke it up. That's how we are going to lose the weight. We are going to break it up into smaller units. Achievable goals. Each week, each unit, each 21-days, will lead you to accomplishing the larger goal.

Small steps. It's magic. I'm telling you.

Small steps will transform your life.

There is a saying, *"It takes one month to recover, repair or heal your health for every year you have been ill or off-track."* If that is true, it would take a minimum of five months for a person to reclaim their health if they were sick for five years.

Does this "formula" or "saying" work for everyone? Of course not! Nothing works for everyone.

However, I agree with this saying. I have seen it work over and over in my practice. It's just a saying that means transformation takes time. This book is about transforming your health. Losing weight will not solve all your health problems but losing weight significantly improves health.

Decide to change. Then figure out the "why"? *What are you fighting for?* Then start immediately. Don't think about five years or five months. Put your blinders on and start the initial 21-day phase.

How much weight can you lose in 21 Days?

I don't know.

Bryan L. lost 26 pounds in 21 days in a *Quantum Paleo Diet Competition* I did with a company in NYC, in March of 2011.

L. B. lost 21.9 pounds and Sage G. lost 14.9 pounds with the same group.

Group settings are highly effective. Sometimes the results will be magnified when you set up a friendly competition. You may want to get a few people at work, school, or form two teams among your family and friends and then compete for 21 days.

It takes 21 days to form a habit. You can always repeat the rounds. Take a few days off and bring it on again. You can lose any amount of weight, even 100 pounds if you break it up into small pieces.

Decide what you are fighting for. Decide what is worth striving for. Then climb into the ring and get started.

Round 7
The Fight Plan

"That's it?"

I think I should have named this section… "That's It!" When I tell people the diet, they always ask, "Is that it?"

The instructions for the diet is to eat the foods you <u>should</u> eat and avoid the foods you <u>shouldn't</u> eat.

Why?

The recommended or allowed foods have been available for over two million years. During that time we became genetically adapted to eating, digesting and utilizing this type of nutrition. Only in the last 10,000 years did humans start to eat grains, beans, sugar and develop herds of milk-producing livestock. From an evolutionary perspective, it has been a relatively short period of time that we have been eating grains, sugar and legumes, and drinking another species milk on a consistent basis. These foods are so "new" to humans and not everyone can digest them adequately. This is precisely why we have health problems when we ingest grains, beans, dairy and sugar to such a large extent. Our bodies are not designed to eat these foods in our everyday diet and therefore, this can lead to numerous health problems.

Think about it. What if you decided to feed your family dog fast food, pizza, beer, ice cream, bagels, pancakes, potato chips and peanut butter sandwiches? Would you expect your dog to have poor health? Actually, this is probably a bad example. The family dog has been domesticated. It is already eating foods that are processed, from a can, and far removed from its original ancestral diet. In fact, some people already feed their dog these type of foods! A better example would be to take a wild animal that is already eating its natural diet and then forcing it to eat foods that are not part of its genetic blueprint. This cruel experiment would result in an animal that suffers from poor health. Not only that, but you would see poor health pass down to this animals offspring, too. In other words, the results of a poor diet can affect future generations. (Pottenger, Francis M., Elaine Pottenger, and Robert T. Pottenger. *Pottenger's Cats: A Study in Nutrition.*)

The Diet

It's not complicated.

Here it is.

Are you ready?

The diet consists of proteins, vegetables, nuts and seeds, some fruit, lots of healthy fats, little starch, no dairy and zero sugar!

That's it. Grains and legumes are not on the diet.

Let's do one day together right now.

Wake up (Recommended)

Meal 1: Protein/Fat/Coffee/Tea/Fruit (8:00 a.m.)

Example: two-egg omelet with mushrooms, onions, avocado, and one diced turkey sausage. Espresso or Tea. Sliced apple on the side.

Meal 2: Protein/Veggies/Salad (12 noon)

Example: salad with grilled chicken, olive oil and vinegar, olives.

Meal 3: Snack (4:00 p.m.)

Example: celery or carrot sticks with organic almond butter, 1-2 tablespoons. Or a hardboiled egg and a small apple.

Meal 4: Protein/Veggies/Fat/Little Starch (7:30 p.m.)

Example: grilled chicken, fish or meat with vegetables, salad (oil and vinegar), half a yam.

Optional snacks times:

Mid-morning:

I have worked with many people that really do well with a mid-morning snack. This would consist of a little protein and fat. For example, leftover protein from the previous night's dinner. With a little slice of avocado. Or, 10-12 raw almonds and some carrot sticks.

Late night:

If you are still awake four hours after your evening meal, please have another healthy snack.

That's it!

How do you add variety? How do you make it interesting?

There are some great Paleo cookbooks that are available. I listed some in the last chapter called: Resources.

I also put a link to an online Paleo Recipe Cookbook, with over a hundred recipes on my http://PaleoXFit.com site. This recipe ebook has breakfast, lunches, dinners, snacks and even desserts.

If you are serious about losing weight then I want you to get a fairly accurate estimate of how many calories you are consuming on a daily basis. In the section called Round 4 "Tale of the tape," I discussed the need to keep track of your daily caloric intake for at least a week, but preferably the whole 21 days. If you visit my website, http://paleosoul.com in the "Tool" section across the top of the header, there is a daily caloric intake calendar that you should use. This will give you a 'ballpark' number of the approximate "daily caloric intake" you should consume to lose weight either slowly or rapidly. Remember, it's only a tool. Everyone is different and you may have to modify your "math" in order to meet your goals.

Below, I have included two versions of my "one page diet breakdown" that I hand out at workshops. One is for someone that is averaging 1300 calories per day for the first 21 days. The second version is for someone who is larger.

1300 Calorie Plan

Meal 1: Protein + Fruit

One egg, apple, orange, pear, or berries. Espresso or tea.

Calories: 220

Meal 2: Protein + Veggies

Small salad with chicken or salmon plus veggies. Oil and vinegar. Avocado, olives.

No bread, croutons, or cheese.

Calories: 350

Meal 3: Snack—Protein + Fruit or Shake.

One hardboiled eggs plus carrots

or

One tbsp. almond butter with carrot or celery sticks

or

1/8 lb. of sliced turkey with ¼ avocado

or

Eleven cashews and an apple

Calories: 210

Meal 4: Protein + Veggies

4 oz of meat, fish or chicken, duck, etc., veggies

Calories: 300

Meal 5: Snack

Two medium hardboiled eggs (optional, can be inserted mid morning or late night)

Calories: 140

Total Calories: 1220 (This is well under 1300 calories and will leave room for larger portions)

When someone is doing the 21-day *Quantum Paleo* program, I like to see my patient initially eat five meals per day. Eating more often during this phase will help your metabolism get more efficient and you won't feel hungry all the time. Later on you can transition to four meals per day if you prefer. Some experienced "Paleo Experts" will eat 3-4 times per day. This is a great idea for them, but as a beginner I would like you to follow my advice. If you are hungry all the time and lose your enthusiasm than nobody wins.

Now here is the 1900 plan.

1900 Calorie Plan

Meal 1: Protein + Fruit

> Three eggs, apple, orange, pear, or berries. Coffee or tea.

> Calories: 400

Meal 2: Protein + Veggies

> Salad with chicken or salmon plus veggies. Oil and vinegar. Avocado, olives.

> No bread, croutons, or cheese.

> Calories: 400

Meal 3: Snack—Protein + fruit or shake.

> Two hardboiled eggs plus carrots

> or

> almond butter with carrot or celery sticks

> or

> ¼ lb. of turkey with ¼ avocado

> or

> 15 cashews and apple

Calories: 300

Meal 4: Protein + Veggies

6 oz of meat, fish, chicken, duck, etc., veggies

Calories: 400

Meal 5: Snack (see meal 4).

(Optional, may be inserted mid morning or late night if still awake.)

Calories: 300

Total Calories: 1800 (We are 100 calories under, leaving room for error on calculations)

Summary:

The calorie counting is only for those that have a big weight loss goal. If you are serious about losing weight, especially in the initial 21 days, then it is imperative that you weigh yourself and track your food. If you are simply doing this for maintenance and a slow transformation of health and body composition, then there is no need to track your caloric intake.

What if you go to my calculations page and the calculator says you should be at 1500 calories per day? Then divide 1500 calories by four meals and you will realize that you will have to eat an average of 375 calories per meal on a four meal a day schedule. If you choose to eat five meals per day, then you can average 300 calories per meal. It's math. It's really simple.

Once you do your math the first time it becomes easy. Repeat the routine for 21 days. I want you to put a little effort into this. When you take responsibility for your own "math" you will begin to master your body. Just do it. It's worth it.

Most of my patients will use a free online and mobile app tool, like http://myfitnesspal.com . It is easier to set up your "profile" on your desktop or laptop rather than setting it up on the mobile App. After you set up your "profile" and create a username and password, download the free mobile "My Fitness Pal" app for daily updating and to stay connected at each meal. The app will also show you at any given moment during the day how many calories you have left to eat. Other sites have similar programs so feel free to find the best one for you.

You don't have to use "MyFitnessPal" forever. I recommend you start using it immediately and continue using it until you are not in any jeopardy of "falling off the wagon". The software will update your "math" at each meal, and prevent self-sabotaging which is the number one reason that people fail in any diet program.

Flying By The Seat of Your Pantry

This section was named and co-written by my wife, Rachel. Rachel is a classically trained Chef who has her own "Cooking School" and popular food blog called **Food Fix** (http://www.food-fix.com). Rachel has also competed and kicked butt on the popular Food Network cooking competition show: *Chopped!* If you want to see Chef Rachel compete on television, she will be in the "Christmas/Holiday Episode of *Chopped!*, on the Food Network airing in December of 2012. Sign up for her Food Blog and get the exact air date when it gets released by the Food Network. Rachel's recipes are often featured by ABCnews.com, too.

Cooking for yourself at home, is a good thing on many levels. For our purposes it is especially useful because it will allow you to control what you eat, the quality of the ingredients and how it's prepared. You'll rely less on take-out, and processed foods that usually contain hidden calories, and occasionally hidden grains, sugar, chemicals, artificial coloring and additives, as well as exceedingly high levels of sodium.

Here are some key ingredients and pantry items you'll want to keep on hand so you can pull together some of the simple meals and recipes that you will find in many of the Paleo cookbooks (see the **Resources** section for cookbook suggestions).

Herbs

Fresh herbs will remain fresh and keep for up to a week if wrapped loosely in a damp paper towel and stored in an airtight zipper bag or plastic container. This is an especially good way to store herbs with delicate leaves, like cilantro, basil and tarragon. Another way to keep hardier herbs fresh is treat them like fresh flowers and put them in water, in a vase and keep them in the fridge. They are easier to access this way and give you a nice bright "green" bouquet to look at each time you open the fridge.

Spices

Basics to keep on hand: cumin, garlic powder, onion powder, cayenne, red pepper flakes, curry powder, chile powder, dried thyme, dried oregano, coriander, Chinese five spice, ras al hanout, cinnamon, allspice, cloves, vanilla extract, smoked paprika, sweet paprika, cardamon, mustard powder and black pepper. Hot sauces like Tabasco and Siracha are good to have on hand as well.

Yes, whole spices, ground fresh for each application are the best way to get the most flavor. If you have the time, the grinder and the inclination to go this extra mile, go for it. Let's be real! Pre-ground and packaged spices are just fine! Just buy small quantities and try to replenish spices that have been laying around more than six months. Use a sharpie to mark them with the date so you know when they've lost their peak of flavor and need to be replaced.

Fats and Oils

Low-fat diets have become as antiquated as the ads that show doctors telling us that smoking cigarettes are good for the digestion. What remains true is that our bodies need fat. Fat makes everything taste and feel better in your mouth. Fat also helps satiate our appetites. In other words, eating quality fat at every meal will keep you from being hungry all the time. Not all fats are good for you.

Here's the lowdown on oils you should eat:

High quality, flavorful oils made from nuts (almond, hazelnut, walnut, macadamia), avocado oil, and more expensive extra virgin olive oils should be used for drizzling, flavoring, or dressing foods, but not for cooking.

For medium heat sautéing or browning food, use less expensive extra virgin olive oils. For high heat cooking you can use coconut oil, clarified butter (ghee), or unprocessed palm oil.

Note: *Oils you don't use every day, especially delicate*

nut oils, should be kept refrigerated. When you want to use them, run the bottle under warm water to partially "melt" if they become solid in the fridge.

Avoid canola, safflower, sunflower, soybean, grape seed, cottonseed, or other "vegetable oils," margarine, or any other hydrogenated oils.

Note: *Clarified butter/Ghee (I do allow this for cooking. You can go online and look up "Ghee" on the Internet to learn more about it.)*

Nuts and Seeds

These make great go-to snacks that will satisfy hunger, provide healthy fats, and give you the crunch and texture factor that many people miss when avoiding grains. Don't overdo these. A small amount goes a long way. Ideally, buy raw nuts and seeds and roast them in your own oven at a low heat (300 degrees) for 8–12 minutes, if you prefer them that way. Chop them, grate them, or grind them into recipes to add fat, flavor, and texture to salads, dressings, coatings/rubs, cut up fruit, sautéed vegetables, or shakes. If possible, keep refrigerated to ensure freshness.

Broths

Vegetable, chicken, or beef broths can now be found in most grocery stores but unless you can find "Organic, Low Sodium, NO MSG" versions, you would be better off passing on this store-bought item and consider making your own and freezing it in pint size containers to use in a pinch to make soups, add moisture to sautéing vegetables, poach proteins, or add flavor to just about anything.

Non-Dairy Milks

These can be high in carbs and calories if you are not careful to buy only "Unsweetened." Avoid soy milk. Opt instead for milks derived from nuts, hemp or coconut milk in cans for cooking, and in the refrigerator section of the grocery store in "milk carton" packaging for use in shakes. You can even find a coconut milk-based creamer for coffee. Again, avoid those non-dairy creamers with sweeteners or artificial sweeteners that are derived from soy and hydrogenated oils. Always avoid high-fructose corn syrup.

Flour Alternatives

Coconut flour, nut meals, or nut flours. Buy in small quantities and keep refrigerated as the oil in nuts can go rancid if left out. These items should last a few months in the fridge.

Sweeteners

Avoid all artificial or so-called "natural" sugar alternatives. You want to train your palette and your "head" to crave less sugar or less intensity of sweetness. Dowsing everything with fake sugar or drinking "diet" drinks may lower the calorie count as compared to using sugar but your brain does not know the difference and will demand its "fix." In moderation, use maple syrup, raw honey, or raw sugar when needed rather than an artificial substitute.

Cheeses/Yogurt/Dairy

For the first 21-Day Round, or until you reach your goal weight, you should avoid cheese and dairy products. No exceptions. Even when you reach your goal weight these should be eaten in moderation and with consideration since they pack a lot of calories and produce a lot of mucus in many people. Milk and cheeses are very hard to handle for many people and do not always promote great health as is popularly believed.

Having said that (after the initial 21 days is completed), I consider cheese a better snack alternative than anything grain-based since it is high in protein and low in carbs and will give you some needed fats in your diet. Dry, aged cheeses, and goat and sheep milk cheeses are a better choice than creamy or processed cheeses made from cow's milk. Choose organic dairy sources whenever possible to avoid hormones and antibiotics. A high-quality, unsweetened yogurt can provide probiotic support for your digestive tract.

A moderate amount (1/4–1/2 cup) of plain low or no-fat yogurt mixed with fruit, nuts or seeds, grated coconut, and some flax oil makes a great treat for breakfast or anytime that can break up the meat and veggie monotony. Many people cannot handle dairy at all. I have the ability to test in my office to see how sensitive my patients are to dairy. If they are getting "zero" reaction to ingesting these foods, I allow it with moderation. If dairy shows up in their lab work as a food sensitivity or food allergy, I have them abstain. Remember, no dairy for the first 21 days!

Milk, cheese, and yogurt are not considered "Paleo" by some Paleo experts. I love Dr. Kurt Harris's blog, http://archevore.com. I really respect his knowledge and information on the subject. Dr. Harris uses heavy cream in his coffee, and even drinks heavy cream for the fat content. He also eats high quality cheeses. Again, we are seeing an array of points of view and opinions on the subject of dairy.

Another blog site that I enjoy and respect is http://drcate.com . She approves of quality dairy as part of a Paleo diet. She points out that anti-dairy research is tainted because they use highly pasteurized dairy for their experiments. Here is an exerpt from her blog.

"None of the animal studies performed by members of the anti-dairy camp use milk in its natural state. Research comparing whole, fresh milk to processed (pasteurized/

homogenized, or dehydrated and reconstituted) shows that animals fed processed milk develop osteoporotic bones, enlarged and fatty livers and hearts, whereas the animals fed fresh milk do not. They conclude that raw milk and processed milk are inherently different products and it follows that they would have different health effects. This is why they recommend consuming unprocessed dairy, in the form of fresh milk, cream, butter, homemade kefir, or raw milk cheese. (Yoghurt is typically made with pasteurized milk.)"

My opinion is zero milk, cheese and yogurt for the first 21 days. Give your body a break. Then either take a food sensitivity test (IgG Food Assay) and learn exactly where you stand with dairy, or use it moderately and see if you truly are doing well eating dairy. (To arrange a Food Sensitivity (IgG) test, go to my website http://TheHealthFixer.com)

Canned/Jar Goods The following items are good in a pinch to add to a salad, dress with a vinaigrette, heat up with some oil and garlic, etc.

Artichoke hearts, hearts of palm, tuna (low sodium), salmon, sardines, anchovies, smoked oysters, nut butters (low or no sugar content, and no trans fats or "natural" style with the oil floating on top), plum tomatoes, whole or diced, salsa, tapenades, olives, roasted peppers, capers, canned fruit packed in natural juices (no syrups), unsweetened applesauce, dried unsweetened fruits (apricots, dates, raisins, cranberries are okay in moderation) and yams (not packed in syrup or if packed in syrup, well rinsed).

Note: *most vegetables should not be eaten from cans because they are over cooked and processed with preservatives and sodium. Frozen is a better choice for vegetables that you want to have on hand and/or store. Your best bet for flavor and nutrition is to use fresh vegetables, blanched, steamed, sautéed, or roasted.*

A Word On Buying Meats and Fish

The *Quantum Paleo* lifestyle has you eating more meats, fish, eggs, poultry and therefore you may want to give a thought to the quality of these proteins you will consume. Strictly eating organic meats can be expensive and even hard to find, though with consumer support and changing attitudes in this country they are more accessible than ever.

Farmer's markets are more prevalent than ever and there is usually a meat and poultry farm represented at these venues. If you can't find, or can't afford, 100% organic meats and poultry, then the next best alternative is to buy those marked "hormone-free," antibiotic-free," "cage-free" or "grass-fed." These can be found in almost any supermarket these days and most certainly at national chains like Whole Foods or Trader Joe's type of stores.

As far as fish goes, here is a link to Monterey Bay Aquarium's seafood watch. They post the dos and don'ts for buying seafood that is safe and sustainable. It is a good site to bookmark and check back with every so often, because it does get updated and conditions change.

http://www.montereybayaquarium.org/cr/seafoodwatch.aspx

Planning and Preparation Give You the Edge in this Fight!

The *Quantum Paleo* lifestyle allows for plenty of eating. You will not starve! The key to success is feeding your body the foods that will give it the most energy, vitality and balance of "calories-in" to "calories-out". This takes some planning, but it's not that complicated. You are going to be eating 4-5 times a day, so packing snacks and lunch to take to work or for "on the road" will keep you from going hungry and entering the "knock out" zone—this is when you eat anything you can get your hands on because you are starving and lightheaded and your caloric intake for the day gets knocked out of whack.

Here we provide some ideas for everyday eating, some easy, some a little more labor-intensive but worth the time to get some variety and flavor into your meals. There are home-cooked options as well as options you can easily find in a diner, deli, or take-out menu. Cooking for yourself is always going to be the best alternative because home-cooked meals give you control over salt, sugar and fat, which tend to be higher in take-out food. If you spend a few hours on a Sunday, or in the evening, preparing some go-to items to keep in the fridge, you will always be able to throw together a quick and *Quantum Paleo* friendly meal. For example:

Hard boil two dozen eggs, peel and keep in airtight container.

Cooked (grilled, baked, broiled) boneless chicken breasts or thighs

Roasted tomatoes/peppers

Roasted root vegetables

Cooked vegetables (quickly blanched broccoli, asparagus, etc)

Roasted Nuts

Always have on hand:

Baby carrots

Apples, pears, other fruit you like

Celery/salad greens/lettuces

Eggs

Sliced turkey, ham or other meats (not for sandwiches,

but for "roll-ups" or use in salads, to fry up with eggs, etc.)

Hunt and Gather Guide

For making choices on the fly, here is your basic list of YES foods and NO foods:

<u>Yes</u> Foods!

Eggs (learn to eat them without bread!)

Nuts

Seeds

Coconut—yes, in every form (the meat, the milk, the oil)

Coffee/Tea (Try a shot of espresso rather than the old habit of milk and sugar!)

Protein Powders—yes, but avoid soy, choose whey that is hormone free/low carb/low sugar

Beef, pork, poultry, game meats, grass-fed meat, offal, bone marrow, wild caught seafood is preferred

Fruits, vegetables, salad greens

Oils, vinegars, lemon juice (oil as mentioned above)

<u>No</u> Foods!

Whole grains, oatmeal, cornmeal, etc.—no. This

means anything made with flour or other grains. Bread, pasta, cake, bagels, cereals, breading on fried foods, etc.

Beans and legumes

Artificial sweeteners—avoid. They train you to crave sweets and they are not healthy choices.

Juices—as a beverage NO. Too much sugar and calories. But OK to use as a flavor enhancer in a dressing or marinade.

Sugar

Say, "No" to dairy, cheese, yogurt, for the first 21 days.

Occasionally!

Dark chocolate, 60% cacao and above

Red wine

Cheeses—in moderation they are acceptable. Hard aged cheeses best choice. (After 21 days, and only if you can handle dairy.)

Yams and sweet potatoes—occasionally. Not every meal

Potatoes

A Word About Meal Labels and Habits

We live with the labels "Breakfast," "Lunch," "Dinner," and "Snack." Each one of these immediately conjures up a list of acceptable foods that make up our version of what those meals should be. Do you have absolutes about what is a "normal" breakfast, lunch, dinner, or snack? Are there meal configurations that you are stuck with?

The American diet dictates eggs, bread, smoked meats, cereals, pastries and fruit for breakfast, sandwiches, and sandwich variations, burgers, fries, salads for lunch, and a big meat, potatoes, vegetable and dessert for dinner. Snacks are crunchy chips or pretzels that come out of a bag or candy bars.

The *Quantum Paleo* lifestyle asks you to step outside these parameters and look at meals more flexibly and to retrain your daily meal habits. I hear people box themselves into high-calorie, weight gaining corners by saying things like:

"I can't eat eggs without bread."

"I need something sweet for breakfast."

"A meal isn't complete without a starch."

"I'm a meat and potatoes guy when it comes to dinner."

"I can't live without pasta a few times a week."

"I can't stand water, I have to drink something sweet with my meal."

Try mixing it up a bit. Eat hardboiled eggs as a snack instead of as a breakfast only item. Eat last night's dinner leftovers for breakfast. A bowl of fruit, yogurt and nuts can be dinner. Finish dinner with a piece of hard cheese and an apple instead of the "needed" sweet and see how satisfying it can be (after 21-days). Make a small salad with nuts and unsweetened dried fruit a mid-morning snack and you won't get the burn and crash you would get from a candy bar or high-carb chip.

Being a Victor, Not a Victim

Quantum Paleo is an eating plan, but it's more than that. You will not succeed unless you can become clear about what you are fighting for and that you are willing to fight for it. Whatever it is, it's got to be strong enough for you to fight and win, to be the VICTOR over the habits, excuses, temptations and status quo of the everyday American diet and the barrage of bad choices available to you.

Reaching your weight and health goals will be

determined by making the choice to be a VICTOR with this mentality:

"I eat foods that I know will contribute to my goals."

"I don't eat foods I know will be detrimental to my health and my goals."

"I make choices that support my well-being."

"I am in charge. If I eat something not on the plan, I get back on the plan with my next meal."

"I deserve great health, a killer body, longevity, vitality, energy and a clear mind. I can achieve this with my diet and lifestyle."

"I accept eating well, as a powerful lifestyle that gives me control over my eating, health and waist size."

"I enjoy great, high-quality foods. I am the master of my health and vitality destiny."

You are giving away your power and acting like a VICTIM if you hear yourself saying:

"I can't help eating cake, candy, etc. because my office is always having some birthday or other occasion where people are bringing in treats."

"My lifestyle/work/schedule doesn't allow me to eat healthy or well."

"I have no time to eat well. I'm always on the go."

"I would eat better if it weren't for my kids, husband, or wife, who insist on bad foods in the house, etc."

"Someday, when the timing and circumstances are right, I'll be able to eat better."

P.S. on dairy

After the 21-day initial phase is completed, you will need to make a decision on where you stand with dairy. If you completely eliminated milk, cheese, and yogurt, then when you reintroduce dairy you may see a reaction. You may have symptoms of intestinal gas, flatulence and mild gastritis (stomach ache). You may have excessive amounts of mucus in your throat, nose and sinuses, or you may see a change in your stool. Dairy is a problem for you, if you have any reaction. Another way to assess the situation is to perform the Food Sensitivity (IgG) Test that I mentioned earlier. This test will tell you if milk, cheese, yogurt and eggs are an issue. It will also tell you if grains and a total of 96 different foods are reacting in a negative way in your body. Learn more about this test at my website: TheHealthFixer.com

Which of the three categories do you fit into?

Those that can eat dairy with no issues.

Those that can never eat dairy: no exceptions.

Those that can tolerate certain types of dairy, in certain quantities and at certain frequencies.

It will take some work, trial and error, and possibly a blood test to determine if you have food intolerances. It is my opinion that less than 40% of people on the planet have absolutely zero issues with dairy. Are you one of them?

Round 8
The Post-Fight

Staying in the Pocket!

Getting in the pocket, zone, or groove. Hitting the sweet spot. I use these sayings to describe when someone is in their optimal state of health. When everything is working correctly in the body and the person's health is predictable and consistent.

My practice attracts patients that want to get into the pocket. I am not a medical doctor. I don't specialize in handling a health crisis, or diagnosing, managing or treating disease. I am really good at getting people into their pocket, zone, or groove regarding their health.

First, I listen to the story of how they got into their present situation. This always reveals a few clues. I usually incorporate some kinesiology/muscle testing that helps me prioritizes and identify the hidden or underlying trouble spots. Then I look for simple and common sense solutions to get people back on track. I look at diet, nutrition, lifestyle, emotional balance and all the health basics. Then I set them up on a comprehensive program to build back their health. This is very similar to meeting with a personal trainer with the goal of getting your physical body into shape. My approach is to work from the inside out. That is why I call it "health fixing" rather than "disease fixing."

"As you build health, you become less sick!"

"Sickness doesn't exist when you are living in the pocket!"

"Disease fixing" is identifying the microbe, infection, organ, or system that is malfunctioning and then setting up a medication plan to treat and manage those symptoms. Most medications, by design, are produced to manage and treat symptoms, not to actually cure the disease or ailment. Therefore, you may need to take the longer, less travelled path if you really want to cure something.

My hands are tied. I am not allowed to carry a prescription pad. It forces me to think differently. "How can I build this person's health? What would be the one or two areas that would strengthen the whole person if we could make progress in that department?" It forces me to look for the cause and rehabilitate the person's health from the ground floor up.

You may think this is too simple. It is not enough. I would venture to say that at least 60-75% of people whose health has crumbled, originally did it to themselves either knowingly or unknowingly. There are exceptions to this hypothesis. Yes, Lance Armstrong got cancer as an elite athlete. Yes, we all know people with genetic diseases. Take a look at the Top 10 Causes of death in the United States today, according to the Center of Disease Control (CDC). Genetic disease does not show up.

Number of deaths: for leading causes of death

- Heart disease: 616,067

- Cancer: 562,875

- Stroke (cerebrovascular diseases): 135,952

- Chronic lower respiratory diseases: 127,924

- Accidents (unintentional injuries): 123,706

- Alzheimer's disease: 74,632

- Diabetes: 71,382

- Influenza and Pneumonia: 52,717

- Nephritis, nephrotic syndrome, and nephrosis: 46,448

- Septicemia: 34,828

- Source: Top Causes of Death in the US (Center for Disease Control)

Heart disease, at number one, is thought to be largely preventable with diet and lifestyle. Cancer can go either way. Yes, some people get cancer for clearly unknown reasons. Others can get cancer because of exposure to chemicals, toxins, radiation and other external agents. Some of these hazardous substances could have been avoided through better education. Some people treat their body poorly. They smoke, drink, eat foods saturated with chemicals and succumb to diseases associated with this type of exposure.

Do you realize that we eat food that is exposed to chemicals, poisons and sometimes radiation (radiating processed meats is now a common technique to kill bacteria and increase shelf-life). Sound harsh? Think about it. Vegetables are sprayed with chemicals and pesticides. What about animal protein and fish? The major food manufacturers are not interested in your health and well-being. That is why I always recommend buying your meat and fish as natural and wild as possible. Did you know that these poisons disrupt your hormonal balance? Many are also carcinogens.

Can eating better quality foods, avoiding grains, legumes and sugar, minimizing exposure to harmful toxins and exercising consistently truly lead to better health? Of course!

One of my favorite things to do is have my patients start a 21-day eating regimen that includes a kit of herbs to cleanse the body. This restarts your body's "computer," and is the fastest way to get you back in the pocket. It's a whole program called the Purification Diet. I now combine it with *Quantum Paleo*, and call it *Paleo Purification Program* or *Paleo Detox*.

When patients get into their pocket or groove, their lab work often improves dramatically. Their vitality and libido improves. The immune system strengthens. Other areas that improve are: hormonal balance, memory, sleep, digestion, bowel movement and function as well as the health of the hair, skin and nails.

I had a professor that told us to remind our patients that it typically takes one month to heal for every year you have been "out of the pocket" (in a state of less than optimal health). Let's say, that you have not been well for three years. Then according to this formula, it would take a minimum of three months to turn your health around.

I have seen many people push their recovery at a faster pace if they begin their journey with our *Paleo Purification Program*. Of course, some people are dealing with chronic illness. I have seen patients with chronic illness and disease build their health to such amazing levels, often to the point that their disease plays a minor role in their lives. That would definitely be a worthy goal and something *worth fighting for*, too.

The Ninja Mind keeps the weight off

It takes a certain mindset to keep the weight off. It doesn't come easy for most people. It is not something you are born with. It needs to be studied, and then practiced. It requires mastery.

For me it is a constant struggle. I am on the path. My stepdad George is a 'black belt' in self-control with regards to the refrigerator. He says, "The mouth is in lockdown at 8 p.m." That's it. You cannot get more food into him when he decides he is finished. Chocolate torture, wine torture, nothing! I can be persuaded pretty easily. Well, not these days, but most of my adult life. A light twist of the arm and I'm yelling "Uncle." Then I will eat sweets or have a beer. That is the 'old' me. The 'new' me practices "The Ninja Mind Set."

My friend Daryl pours some water on his food when he is done eating at a restaurant. Have the waiter remove your plate when you first feel satiated, this way you don't keep picking at the food until it is completely consumed. There are a lot of tricks and tips. Brushing your teeth immediately after eating. Have you tried that one?

My advice focuses more on the mindset and philosophy, rather than tricks and tips.

The big question is:

"How do you bridge the gap between discipline and will power?"

I wish I were the perfect role model so I could tell you the most enlightened way to do it. I'm not. I am the teacher, but I am also the student. As the student I have struggled. I have found that there is actually no technique that can close that last little gap between sticking to "The Plan" and wanting a freakin' piece of chocolate.

Today was a great example. This afternoon I took myself to this great little place around the corner from my office on Twentieth and Broadway. It's owned by the celebrity, Chef Tom Colicchio. Chef Tom hosts the hit television show "Top Chef" and owns several fine dining restaurants in addition to his little sandwich/ bistro place "Wich' Craft." They have great coffee and they also have a double stacked chocolate chip cookie with cream filling. It is built like an Oreo cookie but much bigger.

In the past, my routine would be to go to the store, every afternoon, and get a coffee and a double cookie. These days I'm committed to staying on track. I still crave an afternoon coffee and cookie. What a dilemma!

Back to the story of struggle, torture, suffering, and self-flagellation:

I'm at the counter. They recognize me as the coffee and cookie guy. This is not a good sign when a local store recognizes you as a longtime cookie customer. Especially when I stopped ordering cookies for over a year at this point. My legacy has remained intact! I say, "Small coffee please".

She says, "Would you like the double cookie today?"

Augghhhhhhhhhhhh! I'm going into DTs. Delirium Tremors. Google this if you don't know the term. It is what alcoholics and drug addicts get when they are suffering physiological withdrawals.

I wonder if she can see that I'm really chewing this question in my head like a stale piece of gum. Can you picture the carnival wheel in the television show 'Wheel of Fortune'? I can see that same wheel spinning in my head. On my mind's 'Wheel' I have pictures of a cookie, cookie + coffee, an empty plate, a peanut butter and jelly sandwich, a piece of chocolate, a bowl of ice cream, a turkey sandwich, slice of pizza, a beer, hamburger and fries … you get the idea? Also on this wheel is a picture of my 'fat unhealthy self,' and my "lean happy self." I came to the store with my 'Wheel' set on Coffee-Only. The counter person just gave my wheel a big spin. This is probably 15 months since I even ordered a cookie! Now I'm obsessing about all my choices. I want it to land on 'cookie' (Double cookie, actually).

I grab the "wheel" with all my strength. I force it to stop on *small coffee*.

I hear myself say the words, "No, thank you!"

She said, "Would you like our Chocolate Brownie instead?" She gives the wheel another big ole' spin!

Augghhhhhhhhhhhhhhhhhhhhhh!

Can't she see that I'm weak? My willpower is draining fast. I may actually faint.

"No, thank you. Just the coffee, please."

I grab the wheel. Stop it on *small coffee.*

Pay for the coffee. Leave the store in a cold sweat!

So, what happened? Let's review.

What happened is I still suffer. I really do. Maybe you won't, but I do.

So, what's different?

I really have a strong … *What are you fighting for?* at this time in my life.

Two categories motivate me: my health, and wanting to look my best. Not necessarily in that order! (Smiling)

My commitment to *What I am fighting for* is bigger than my weakness for a double chocolate chip cookie, or a slice of pizza, or a bowl of ice cream every night.

Anthony Robbins, the author and motivational speaker, wrote (I'm paraphrasing here) that "you need to decide which is more painful: the pain of not having temporary satisfaction or instant gratification (the cookie), versus the pain of not reaching your long-term goals" (getting healthy, looking good, etc.).

So there is the rub! In the past I have chosen the instant gratification rather than the long-term solution. Now, more and more, I am making better choices. Having a strong *"what are you fighting for?"* that you update on a regular basis allows you to live your life with the big picture in mind.

Think about it; there is no way to bridge the gap between discipline and will power, with gimmicks or tricks. I guess there are always drugs. Yes, drugs are a possible solution. Amphetamines or stimulants are highly addictive and cause an extreme load of stress on your heart and nervous system. It is too dangerous to get your "discipline" in a pill or a potion.

First off, decide *what you are fighting for*. Then get motivated for 21 days and do Round 1 of *Quantum Paleo* with all your heart. Get in the habit of eating smaller meals 4-5 times per day. Get in the habit of exercising 4-6 days per week. Start to learn and practice making choices that will help you in the long run. When the first Round of 21 days is complete, take two or three days off and do another Round. Then take a few more days off and do another round. By this time you will have developed enough strength to maintain your goals. Always read and update your *What are you fighting for?* index card.

The more solid you are with the *What are you fighting for?* **the easier it will be to stay on track.**

"This is my job"

That needs to be your answer to the following questions:

"How did you lose weight?"

"How do you stay in shape?"

"How do you get up and workout before work?"

"How do you do it?"

I want you to start interacting with being healthy and being fit as if it was your job. It's your job to stay healthy. Isn't that true for you? It has to be. You can't "f" around with this! It is a life or death situation. You don't have to have a heart attack to get inspired. Actually, your ticket has already been issued in your name with heart attack, Type 2 diabetes and debilitating degenerative diseases written in the subject line. The only thing that you can edit is "when" and "what if." Everyone has the potential to succumb to disease and infirmity. Tear up the "ticket." Refuse to give in.

What if you make it your priority to live healthy, eat healthy and exercise consistently with passion? If you choose to make it the highest priority, you can potentially change the "when" or the "expiration date" on your life line. Instead of falling apart before your time, choose to live long and age with strength, stamina and great health.

I don't know about you, but when the alarm rings on workdays, I just get up immediately. The alarm rings and I get up. I don't discuss with myself about the possibility about not going to work that day. Why?

I have a "relationship" with my work that is not negotiable. I go into work and do my job. Period. My family needs me. I need food and shelter. It's a matter of survival.

Health has to be the same way.

Raise the stakes. Make it extremely important. That's the trick. That is all you need to know.

With that one realization you will take the responsibility of staying well to the highest level.

"I stay healthy because it's my job!"

What will it cost you to let yourself gain the weight back?

If you decide that this is your job, then it is worth putting into your schedule. A job comes with a schedule. I used to work out when I had some free time. That is planning for failure. As a result, I was overweight, fatigued, depressed and starting to have health problems.

Since 2009, I book workouts into my schedule every week. Start doing this. It works.

Monday, Tuesday, Thursday, and Friday I'm at Hell's Kitchen CrossFit from 7:00–8:00 a.m. I see my first patients at 9:00 a.m. I get up at 4:45 a.m. to catch a 5:30 a.m. bus to NYC. Door to door it takes me 90 minutes.

I also do 3 spin classes per week on my lunch break. Then I go to a gym near my house on either Saturday or Sunday with my daughter and do a light workout, stretch and some cardio. Otherwise, I take long walks with my wife and dogs on the weekends.

This is my job. I just do it. I schedule it and get it done. I don't consider if I'm in the mood or not. That's irrelevant. It's not my hobby. It's on my schedule. It needs to get done. It's my freakin' job.

As soon as you begin the journey and start to chisel off the debris revealing the body that you want to live in, you must take on this new attitude.

"Of course I exercise."

"Of course I choose healthy foods."

It's what we do!

How To Get Off the Roller-Coaster!

I have done quite a bit of gaining and losing weight throughout my adult life. This is often called the "roller-coaster." Have you heard that most people lose weight and then gain the weight back? Sometimes they regain more weight then their original starting weight.

This is going to be a short segment.

There are just two solutions.

Solution #1: *What are you fighting for?*

You really need to have the "why" not only figured out, but written down. It becomes more powerfully embedded in your mind when you write it down and read it often. Then when you tell others your goals, it picks up momentum. Tell someone you love that your goal is to keep the weight off. The 'why' is even more important than simply sharing a numerical value. Tell your friend or loved one, that the reason I will keep the weight off is _____.

"I will keep the weight off because I want to be able to play with my grandkids!"

"I will keep the weight off because I want to look

amazing in a bathing suit each and every decade of my life!"

"I will keep the weight off and continue to eat healthy and exercise because I want to have a healthy heart!"

Solution #2: Exercise!

Over the years, whenever I work with patients that lose weight without adopting an exercise program, I worry.

I worry because you are about 75% more likely to gain back the weight if you have not made exercise part of your life.

Conversely, we can safely say that you are 75% more likely to keep off the weight if you have a vigorous, consistent and frequent exercise program as part of your daily or weekly regimen.

That's it. Don't make it harder than that.

Make it a life or death commitment. Because it is!

The Acceptable Window

Everyone's weight vacillates throughout the day. Mine can fluctuate three to four pounds. I may wake up in the morning and my weight is 187 pounds, for example, and then if I weigh myself before bedtime my weight may be 189 pounds. Then the next morning it may be 186.8 pounds and so on.

This is one type of window. It's the window your weight fluctuates throughout the day. This is the daily fluctuation.

The second window is what I call the "Acceptable Window" or "The Allowable Window." The "Acceptable Window" is the most recent average weekly fluctuation of your body weight.

Let's say you started at 176 pounds and after doing the *Quantum Paleo* program for three months you now weigh 150 pounds. My goal for you, and I hope it is your goal too, is to maintain your results. No relapse! Therefore, I want you to understand the weekly fluctuation and learn how to use it.

Here is what I mean. Let's make up a factitious person named Joe Wyndoe who we will use to make the math example more real.

Let's say we had the opportunity to have weighed Joe Wyndoe every day for a week before he started the *Quantum Paleo* program.

***Every weigh-in would be taken first thing in the morning, naked, after your morning urination, moments after arising.

His numbers may have looked like this:

Monday	175.0 lbs.
Tuesday	176.4 lbs.
Wednesday	174.9 lbs.
Thursday	174.7 lbs.
Friday	174.1 lbs.
Saturday	177.4 lbs.
Sunday	177.9 lbs.

The average would be 175.77 pounds. The average is a good number to know, but the weekly window of fluctuation is more important to use as a tool to keep your weight stable.

It's important to know your window of fluctuation. Joe Wyndoe's weight fluctuated between 174.1 to 177.9, which is 3.8 pounds over the course of one week.

Before we go further, I want to add that I also like to know the percent body fat at each window. For the example above, let's say his average was 21.5 % body fat.

Three months on the *Quantum Paleo* program and Joe Wyndoe loses about 25 pounds! Remember weight fluctuates daily. Joe Wyndoe needs to learn his new window of fluctuation. We track him again and find his weight now moves between 149 and 151.5 in a given week. His body fat percent is around 15.5%. Good job!

Joe really wants to maintain his 'new' weight. In the past he always gained the weight back. This time he learns that his 'new' weight will naturally go through a range of 149-151.5 lbs. He loves the way his body looks at this weight. When someone asks his weight. Joe would most likely say that he weighs, "150 pounds".

Joe needs to know his new "window" at this desired body weight and average "body fat %". Joe must fight for his life to keep it! If he sees it start to move up, he needs to take action immediately and fix it. If his window of fluctuation gets up to 152-154 pounds, he should get pissed off. This is not an acceptable window. He needs to immediately analyze his workouts, his food, his bad carbohydrates, his fat intake, his portion size, his sleep, his stress levels and make the necessary modifications to rectify the situation.

Fix it. His math is off. Fix the math!

The only "Acceptable Window" for Joe Wyndoe is 149-151.5 lbs. Period! Fight to stay in your window. Know your window. Fight for it.

CrossFit: The way our bodies were meant to train!

This past year, I switched my training philosophy dramatically. For years, I was always the chest and arms guy, with a little cardio thrown on top. That gave me a decent personal best in the bench press, ample love handles, quite a bit of a belly when I wasn't sucking it in, and mediocre endurance at best.

I can't remember if a patient recommended it to me, or if I stumbled across it on the Internet. Either way, CrossFit training has become my new passion for the past six months.

The following is an article that I pulled from the *CrossFit Journal* website. This article was written by the founder of CrossFit, Greg Glassman, in April of 2002. I couldn't say it better. I would rather quote him and at the same time pay homage to a great innovator of a booming fitness movement.

Foundations (http://journal.crossfit.com/2002/04/ foundations.tpl#featureArticleTitle)

"CrossFit is a core strength and conditioning program. We have designed our program to elicit as broad an

adaptational response as possible. CrossFit is not a specialized fitness program but a deliberate attempt to optimize physical competence in each of ten recognized fitness domains. They are Cardiovascular and Respiratory endurance, Stamina, Strength, Flexibility, Power, Speed, Coordination, Agility, Balance, and Accuracy.

The CrossFit Program was developed to enhance an individual's competency at all physical tasks. Our athletes are trained to perform successfully at multiple, diverse, and randomized physical challenges. This fitness is demanded of military and police personnel, firefighters, and many sports requiring total or complete physical prowess. CrossFit has proven effective in these arenas.

Aside from the breadth or totality of fitness the CrossFit Program seeks, our program is distinctive, if not unique, in its focus on maximizing neuroendocrine response, developing power, cross-training with multiple training modalities, constant training and practice with functional movements, and the development of successful diet strategies.

Our athletes are trained to bike, run, swim, and row at short, middle, and long distances guaranteeing exposure and competency in each of the three main metabolic pathways.

We train our athletes in gymnastics from rudimentary

to advanced movements garnering great capacity at controlling the body both dynamically and statically while maximizing strength to weight ratio and flexibility. We also place a heavy emphasis on Olympic Weightlifting having seen this sport's unique ability to develop an athletes' explosive power, control of external objects, and mastery of critical motor recruitment patterns. And finally we encourage and assist our athletes to explore a variety of sports as a vehicle to express and apply their fitness." Greg Glassman

✳✳✳

After reading Mark Rippetoe and Lon Kilgore's book, called *Starting Strength*, I now know more than ever why multi-joint exercises and functional movement reigns supreme to condition the body.

Rippetoe and Kilgore say that "Physical strength, more than any other thing we possess, still determines the quality and the quantity of our time here in these bodies." As a health provider, my first impulse is to add a few categories to their list, such as, immune system, mental health, etc. But, we could easily miss the point. I know what they mean. They are not saying that other things are not important. Rather, they are examining what is the bare essential to "exist" in "this body" we are inhabiting for the next few decades.

Take a walk through a hospital or a nursing home if you need some insight or motivation. Look at all the people that have lost their strength, they are too weak to walk, sit up in bed, or even feed themselves.

That is one of my biggest fears …

Being trapped in a broken down body!

Possessing physical strength is the foundation of living in the physical world.

The best news is it's something we can all work on.

How many of us know how to get our immune systems in shape? Hopefully, you will learn by reading my blog, but working on our physical bodies is something we can all do.

How many hours per day or per week do you have available to commit to your physical health?

It's a great question.

Because then you need to ask yourself what type of exercise is worth spending your time on.

My daughter Lily, is doing High School Cheerleading.

She is required to do tumbling runs consisting of a double back-handspring followed by a back tuck (flip). Other times she is required to lift and press her teammates into the air. The teammate stands on Lily's hands as she does an overhead press with them.

These are all functional movements, in other words, they require multiple joints working in unison under a load. To revisit, Greg Glassman's quote above about the ten recognized fitness domains *"They are Cardiovascular and Respiratory endurance, Stamina, Strength, Flexibility, Power, Speed, Coordination, Agility, Balance and Accuracy."* That is exactly what is being trained and conditioned in Lily's typical workout.

A bicep curl involves the bending of the elbow to raise the weight. One joint.

A big bicep looks good, but it is not very practical in everyday life. My wrestling coach used to tell us that training the biceps as an isolated exercise was a waste of time. It is not a very important muscle for sports. However, when you go to any gym, that's what people spend an awful lot of time on … bicep curls!

My coach explained that most sports need shoulders, back, butt, trunk, legs, forearms, and grip, and the power that comes from powerful hips and the posterior chain of muscles that run along the back of our bodies. The part we can't see in the mirror!

A 'squat,' which is basically a deep knee-bend with a loaded barbell across your back, involves multiple joints. As you descend into your squat, the hips, back, knees all need to move, as well as multiple muscles need to work in unison to complete the movement.

Multiple-joint exercises train the body the way it was meant to move.

Rippetoe and Kilgore say that "The human body functions as a complete system—it works that way, and it likes to be trained that way. It doesn't like to be separated into its constituent components and then have those components exercised separately, since the strength obtained from training will not be utilized in this way. The general pattern of strength acquisition must be the same as that in which the strength will be used."

They go on to say, "Properly performed, full range-of-motion barbell exercises are essentially the functional expression of human skeletal and muscular anatomy under a load."

What is your goal? If you want to look good, then single-joint exercises will help you meet your goals. If you want to live long, and be able to jump, climb, drag, row, run, skip, thrust, reach, push, pull, bounce, spin, hop, and roll throughout your life, then do exercises that challenge those movements under a load, and start to do functional movements with a load!

At this point you may think, why do I want to do those things anyway?

The inability to do those things defines your physical presence here on the planet. Imagine what it's like to not be able to reach down and pick up your grandkid off the carpet (multiple-joint movement). All those things (run, jump, climb, etc.) are either 'freedoms' or 'limitations.' It's your choice.

That's why I love CrossFit!

The beauty of CrossFit is that it's scalable. Meaning the load and rate of exercise can be varied to meet the age, size, sex, and needs of the individual. If the exercise requires lifting a bar from the floor to an overhead position, then the person can lift a broomstick, or an Olympic barbell with many plates on either end! I can be working side by side in a CrossFit class with an elite athlete. We are doing the same routine. At different weights and different speeds.

What are <u>you</u> fighting for?

That is the question I ask my patients when they are tackling a huge health goal.

What constitutes a huge health goal?

How about losing the weight you accumulated in the past decade? How about balancing your hormones naturally? How about cutting out grains, sugar and dairy, because you know it's time to get your digestion and inflammation under control?

These are goals that pose an extreme challenge because they can't be accomplished over night.

If I can help people get in touch with *What they are fighting for* they will get the springboard they need to launch their quest to transform. What is the one thing that needs to change in order for you to reach your goals?

Deb was referred into my office and wanted to drop 20 pounds.

Why? (I always ask 'why?')

She was getting married in three months. She is 29 years old, and has had this extra weight on her hips, abdomen, thighs and buttocks for her entire adult life. She knew "what" she was fighting for. She now needed a "how". The *Quantum Paleo* program is challenging on its own and I pushed her even harder. I had her do five days per week of cardio. She decided to do three spin classes per week, and two days of walking outside per week. She had been doing one private Pilates class per week which constituted her entire workout regimen. She liked Pilates and I wanted her to continue with that. I wanted her to use the money she was allocating for a "private one-on-one Pilates" session and switch to three Pilates group classes per week. By the way, I don't make people do CrossFit or anything else. Everyone can make their own choices. If I'm asked what I recommend, it is CrossFit. In Deb's case, she loves Pilates and spin classes. Fine.

She worked her butt off. Literally. She lost 23 pounds. At 5'3", that's a huge transformation. That is like a 6'0" tall man losing 40 pounds. Her abs went totally flat. Even sculpted a little. The excess weight on her butt and thighs disappeared! The biggest change was her face went from round, plump and colorless (pallor), to visible classic cheekbones, jaw line and defined collarbones for the first time. Her color was robust, with a natural rosiness due to her invigorated metabolism from diet, exercise and cardio.

Now three months after her wedding, she stabilized her body weight. She actually lost another three pounds since her wedding. She cut back to three to four days per week of cardio and two days of group Pilates. She has wine two nights per week. She doesn't touch bread or pasta during the week, ever. She relaxes on one day of the weekend. Ice cream on Saturday nights only. She doesn't buy it for the house. Her weight will vacillate between 117-120 pounds. That is her "Acceptable Window." If her weight drifts above 120 pounds she immediately gets back on track.

The concept of *What are you fighting for?* is the key to the *Quantum Paleo* program. You must first declare it, and then make it a priority. There has to be a conversation going on in your head. You have to realize that immature voice in your head that doesn't want to work out, that doesn't want to eat healthy, that doesn't want to get off the couch. It is the immature voice of a "four-year-old". Do you want a "four-year-old" to run your life?

My kids are older now. I was lenient in some areas of their life. Sometimes I would let them stay up past their bedtime if we were watching a favorite TV show as a family. When it came to health, education and safety, I became strict. I had the ability to say, "No!"

The same thing happens with my mind. I have a plan to go to the gym.

My "four-year-old mind" says, "Let's skip today."

"NO!" It's not negotiable. Period. "Let's have that cookie now, Daddy." "NO! Eat your protein!"

Deb is getting really good at parenting her "four-year-old" voice. She has ice cream, but not every day. She has wine, but not every day. She is the adult. She decides how to run her life. She has made a decision that she will not allow herself to get above 120 pounds. If or when she does get above 120 pounds, she goes into high alert and makes it a priority to handle it immediately. She will add some more cardio. She will tweak her diet. It is simply not negotiable. Period!

I'm often asked how I teach people to maintain their desired weight. There are tips and tricks but the bottom line is: know "what you are fighting for," then make a pact with yourself that veering from the course is not negotiable. Just like Deb. When you get outside of your "Acceptable Window," it's hammer time!

Round 9
The Fighters

Meet some fighters!

I have been supervising patients making the transition from eating a big grain diet to a Paleolithic type of diet for 14 years. I have seen approximately 1800 patients go through this process. While everyone's experience is different, I chose a handful of cases that will highlight the health potential and possibilities that exist when switching to a *Quantum Paleo* lifestyle.

I cannot tell you the patient's name because there are strict laws against revealing personal information. I changed the cases and names enough to protect the identities. I did not change the patient history, lab values, or the results.

Hormone Helen

"At 51, I hadn't had my period in 11 months. I was suffering from hot flashes every night. After about two months, it escalated to daytime, too. During the day, I could have another six or more hot flashes and a few of those daytime ones would literally soak through my shirt. I started bringing extra shirts to work. I was embarrassed because I knew people would notice a new shirt in the middle of the day. My diet was off when I met Dr. Willen. I gained weight in the last five years and was 17 pounds heavier than I was at 46 years old. That was the age when everything started slipping.

He put me on his program. We just focused on one Round of 21 days at a time. It took me three Rounds of 21 days. Within the first 10 days, my hot flash frequency cut down to nighttime only. Then during my second Round of the *Quantum Paleo* program, I was down to two to three mild hot flashes per week! That's per week, not per day. In my third Round of *Quantum Paleo*, I had one mild hot flash during the entire three weeks!

I have more energy now and my libido returned. I'm sleeping better and getting more total sleep than I have in 10 years. I am making the right choices with my food with very little effort. Dr. Doug told me that exercise would be the stabilizing force, and that is exactly what happened. By making exercise "my job," I am not worried about gaining back the weight. One more thing … I would get a herpes outbreak every few years in the past. Then this past year, it was happening continuously. Dr. Doug said he often sees that sort of thing respond to making the shift towards eating a Paleolithic diet. He's right. That cleared up pretty fast, and I don't feel like it's about to resurface anytime soon. The price of feeling icky is too much, it is now my highest priority to be healthy. It took me all three Rounds but I finally lost 21 pounds total."

Hearty Arty

"I'm 63 years old and have had two stents put in my heart recently. I quit smoking after my heart attack two years ago. I was taking several meds, including meds for my cholesterol, blood pressure, and a blood thinner. Although I cut my weight down 37 pounds already, my cardiologist wanted me to lose at least another 30 pounds. The problem was that my weight hadn't budged in six months.

I decided to do the *Quantum Paleo* program. Dr. Doug suggested I join a CrossFit gym near my office and he put me on the *Quantum Paleo*. I had to stop eating bran muffins, oatmeal, and all the whole grains that the hospital dietician put me on. This made me nervous. I was also scared about all the fat that would be in the *Quantum Paleo* program. Dr. Doug told me the blood tests would prove to me that there was no need to worry. Dr. Doug always tells me, "Fat doesn't make you fat," and "it's the refined carbohydrate diet that is elevating your blood work, not the avocados, eggs and olive oil!"

"I lost an additional 36 pounds on *Quantum Paleo*. It took four rounds of 21 days. The most astonishing thing was that my medical doctor was able to take me off of my blood pressure meds. My statin (cholesterol med) is at the smallest possible dosage, reduced 75%. We decided to leave me on the plavix (blood thinner), because he (cardiologist) feels it's too risky to change that one. I have a 32-inch waist now. Same size as college!"

Jay Pouch

"I had my first colon surgery at the age of 20. After terrible pain, bloating, bloody stools, diarrhea and recurring bouts of fever for two years and numerous hospital visits, my surgeon thought it was time. Over the next 10 years, I needed more surgery. Five more to be exact. Removing about 95% of my large intestine. Eventually they created a "J Pouch." That is where they construct a pouch typically out of the small intestine.

It's also called an ileoanal reservoir procedure. The J Pouch is a storage place for the stool that I eventually pass several times per day.

The reason I came to Dr. Willen, was that at the age of 31 years old, I was still having problems. Digestion, pain, swelling, gas pockets, adhesions, the list goes on. I was on a whole list of medications. Dr. Willen urged me to start the *Quantum Paleo* diet. First he wanted to show me his suspicion of gluten and dairy. He ordered a Food Sensitivity (IgG) Test. In the two weeks that we waited for the results, he had me start on zero grains, zero dairy, and zero sugar. He said if a patient is in a health crisis, they need to be 100% off of the three whites (grains, sugar and dairy). Period. By the time the test came back, I was sleeping through the night. I was reducing my painkillers and anti-inflammatory. I was already feeling better than I had in a long time.

The tests came back with gluten as a big hit. So was dairy and about 10 other foods (food intolerances). All grains were lit-up (positive test findings) in the abnormal ranges. It's now been four months and I really have no symptoms. I was diagnosed with ulcerative colitis, which Dr. Doug said I definitely had. He wanted to know what was causing the ulcerations. He said that grains can do that with some people.

My medical team never felt there was a food

connection. As far as medicine goes, the cause is unknown and it's thought it may be related to some foods, or a problem with the immune system. The funny thing is that for the last 10 years they wanted me to eat a diet of bland foods, including pasta, white bread toast, saltines, noodle soup, etc. I was on a "Neolithic" (agricultural era) diet for the past 10 years. My level of grains was ridiculous! I am so glad I switched from "Neo to Paleo" (Neolithic to Paleolithic)! LOL!!!"

Goode Knight

"Dr. Doug put me on the *Quantum Paleo* program about three months ago. At the time I was sleeping about four total hours per night. I seemed to fall asleep pretty well, but would wake up within one to two hours and then have trouble getting back to sleep. Then eventually I would get to sleep again for another two hours, and then after waking up the second time I wouldn't get back to sleep. I always felt this weird "buzzing" feeling in my body in the middle of the night. It's hard to describe but the best I can do is to say it felt like I had a triple shot of espresso at 2 am every night. I am on zero caffeine by the way.

Dr. Doug explained that all my refined carbohydrates that I was addicted to were hampering my ability to get a good night's sleep. Although he didn't promise anything, he was grinning when he said, "Let's wait and see."

Meanwhile, I needed to lose some weight anyway, and I had a few other things I was dealing with. For example, chronic aches and pains. After about 15 days, I was sleeping through the night. Only about 6.5 hours at first, but then eventually 7.5–8 hours. Dr. Doug suggested that I black out my room and move all electrical things out of the room and start to go to sleep an hour earlier.

I think a big part was getting my health and diet corrected. My aches and pains have reduced 85%. I also lost eight pounds the first three weeks and a total of 22 pounds and maintaining!"

Mike Bladher

"I had been a college basketball player and continued to play in competitive men's leagues throughout my adult life. I ate well, lifted weights and played basketball several times per week. My waist was still 34 inches!

Then at the age of 49, I was taking a leak after watching a movie with my wife and kids and a black looking blood came out with my urine, through the head of my penis. I was very scared. Long story made shorter. A week later I was diagnosed with Bladder Cancer.

Surgery was schedule in a few weeks, big procedure. They were afraid that the cancer was aggressive and already migrated. My prognosis was not good. I went to Dr. Doug to have him look at my diet.

He told me that if he was in my shoes, he would get his diet super cleaned-up before the surgery. He said, "We need to get you in fighting shape." That way you will be the best candidate to create a miracle! He wanted me to eliminate "The 3 Whites: Grains, Dairy and Sugar." I thought my diet was pretty good. He wanted me to go off all flour, grains and totally stop dairy and sugar, too. I had never done this before because I always thought athletes need to eat a lot of healthy grains and several glasses of milk per day. I tried to negotiate with him. I wanted him to allow a little bit of whole grains, and at least a glass of milk every day. He said, "100% compliance" or don't bother starting. I decided to follow the rules. I did the diet perfectly. I approached it like a "fight for my life."

(Note: This story was from 2002. I didn't have the word 'Paleo' in my vocabulary back then. I called it "Getting off of the 3 Whites.")

The surgery went well. My medical team bragged about how fast I recovered. It's been two years now. Cancer free. I still eat this way. I now have a 32-inch waist, play basketball several times per week, and my immune system feels so strong. I never get sick anymore. I sleep like a baby. My allergies have disappeared. I could go on, but I think you get the idea."

(Note: As of January, 2012, Mike is still very healthy, cancer-free and eating a Paleo diet.)

Al Kohol

"I was abusing alcohol for most of my 20's and at 35 years old, it was getting worse. My career and marriage went down the drain. I was 50 pounds overweight and I looked like I was in my late 40s. Alcohol really destroys the skin and ages you rapidly.

I met Dr. Doug after being sober for four weeks. My sponsor in my AA group was a patient of Dr. Doug and he told me to get checked.

Dr. Doug offers all of his patients an opportunity to "Get on Program". This means he gets your diet right, and gives you a routine of daily supplements to address nutritional deficiencies and to build and maintain health naturally. I thought I might benefit from getting on a "health building program" to offset my "destroy my body program" I had been on over the last bunch of years.

I was thinking about having a drink, every day. All day long, actually. I felt like I might slip. I was actually dreaming on most nights that I slipped up and went on a binge again, only to wake up and realize it was only a very vivid dream. I was scared. On top of that I gained another 15 pounds in those first four weeks off of alcohol. I was eating bread, sugar, sweets, desserts, potato chips, pretzels and my favorite was bagels. Bagels for breakfast. Tuna on a bagel at lunch. I was craving bread like an addict.

Dr. Doug put me on the *Quantum Paleo* program. In addition, he did his "weird-arm" testing (nutritional kineseology). This is where he figures out what nutrients and supplements a person needs to reclaim their health. I call it "weird-arm testing" but I have to admit it really works.

Within three days, my sugar cravings were gone. I was off bread. My bloated face and belly started to reduce. Dr. Doug wanted me to do cardio six days per week and weights three times per week. I lost 22 pounds the first month. After three months, I was down 42 pounds. After six months I lost a total of 72 pounds. I was stable in my sobriety. I didn't feel vulnerable to a relapse. I was in a new relationship. I started a new career in a whole new direction. Actually, it was the work I always wanted to do, but never felt confident to pursue it.

Dr. Doug explained to me that getting off of the grains and sugar, in my case, would help tremendously with my addiction. Not only was I addicted to the alcohol, but he said my carbohydrate addiction was 'adding gasoline to the fire'!"

Final Thoughts

"Let others lead small lives, but not you. Let others argue over small things, but not you. Let others cry over small hurts, but not you. Let others leave their future in someone else's hands, but not you."

Jim Rohn

The late Jim Rohn was one of my mentors. I never met him but I listened to his tapes and read his books, over and over again. My final thoughts are woven around two favorite quotes of Jim Rohn, as way to pay homage to this great inspirational teacher.

Losing weight and working on your health can be a catalyst for change in every area of your life. Sometimes we all feel like our life's circumstances are so overwhelming that we don't know where to start. All change starts at a core level. Change the way you eat. Change the way you exercise and your world will change.

Decide what is worth fighting for... and go change your world!

"You cannot change your destination overnight, but you can change your direction overnight." Jim Rohn

Round 10
Wrap Up
Resources

This section will give you a little information on the following:

1. Dr. Doug Willen and how to stay connected.
2. Websites of interest
3. Cookbooks
4. Recommended Reading
5. CrossFit
6. Private phone consults with Dr. Doug
7. Food Sensitivity (IgG) Testing.
8. *"What is Paleo?"* A short book (under 100 pages) also written by Dr. Doug.
9. Information on *Quantum Paleo* weight loss webinars and other future webinar topics.
10. Stay connected with Dr. Doug thru Twitter and Facebook!

About Dr. Doug:

A chiropractor saved me from being "benched" from sports in high school by taking a "hopeless" injury and turning it around. That was my introduction into the power of natural solutions for health. When my family medical doctor could only offer me painkillers and restrictions in reaction to my injury, a local chiropractor offered me solutions! That made a lasting impression on me that ultimately affected my career path. I was a pre-med student at Cornell University when I made a conscious decision to explore alternatives in personal growth and in healthcare instead of moving forward into a conventional medical education. My experience with a chiropractor in high school was one factor in my decision. Another was my long struggle with allergies and my growing disillusionment with the heavy pharmaceutical emphasis of the medical/allopathic model of disease treatment. I worked with alternative practitioners who employed thoughtful investigation into the cause of my allergies, rather than simply treating the symptoms, and helped me with natural solutions in a way that years of shots and drugs could not.

Around The World And Back Home Again.

After college, I traveled extensively in India, Asia, and

Central America living with local people and learning about different cultures, approaches to healthcare and spirituality. It was an invaluable experience that left a lasting impression on me. I returned home, after nearly two years of travel, to pursue my goal of becoming a natural health practitioner. I attended Life University in Atlanta, where I earned my Doctorate in Chiropractic then returned to my home state of New York. After opening a Chiropractic and Nutrition practice in NYC, I started to study with a leader in the field of nutritional kinesiology, Fred Ulan. Dr. Ulan later turned over his New York City practice to me. I was honored to be his protégé and be trusted to take good care of his long-standing patients of many years.

I Take Care Of You The Way You'd Want To Be Taken Care Of.

My business card says "natural solutions for health" and that's what I have always been committed to— finding those solutions and empowering others to take control of and being responsible for their well-being. Since being in practice these past 14 years, I have helped thousands of people regain and rebuild their health through safe, natural supplementation, diet and lifestyle changes and expert chiropractic care. My practice is mostly a "word of mouth" practice because once I take care of people they want their family and friends to come in too. "You're going to love Dr. Doug," is what I strive to have people say to others when they leave my office, and so far, I'm happy to say, they do!

The majority of my patient base are elite level dancers, actors (stage, commercial, television and film), fashion models, musicians, talent agents, producers, casting directors, and wardrobe people from the entertainment industry. My other big group comes from the NYC fashion industry. I take care of the everyday "wear and tear" of dancers that are employed in Broadway shows (Wicked, Lion King, Phantom of the Opera, Billy Elliot, Mama Mia, Memphis, Chicago, etc.) as well as being one of the "go-to specialists" that works with the American Ballet Theater on a daily basis.

We are back in New Jersey again after a brief stint in Brooklyn. My wife, Rachel, is a writer and chef and creator of the popular food blog called, Food-Fix. com. She does Culinary Instruction and private Chef Services and can be contacted through her website. Rachel is also an amazing mom to our two kids, two dogs, and two cats. My son, Max, 23, graduated from The Culinary Institute of America and now he is a chef at the world famous Per Se restaurant in NYC. Per Se is one of only six restaurants in NYC that have all three Michelin Stars. I have always admired my son in many ways, but now that he's 6'5", I really look up to him! My daughter, Lily, 16, is an honor student, great athlete, and loves to spend time with her friends.

Walking The Walk

I'm so lucky to have my practice in New York City where I have access to so many wonderful practitioners. Like many of my patients, I use my body in my work and it's important for me to stay strong and injury free. Regular chiropractic care is essential for me to have longevity in my field and I continue to have personal and professional associations with many fine practitioners. This way, if I can't help you with your health concerns, or I feel they are beyond the scope of my practice, I usually can refer you to someone I respect who can. I belong to CrossFit Hell's Kitchen on Thirty-Sixth Street in NYC. The owner/coach Anthony Preischel has taught me so much in such a short time since I started. The workouts are humbling, reminding me each day that being in shape is a journey and not a destination.

The *Quantum Paleo* program evolved over the last 14 years while working with patients that not only wanted to lose weight, but also wanted to achieve their maximum levels of health and well-being.

I invite you to get involved with this information and not only read, but interact, with the blog community and take action. Now is the time to transform your body, your health, and your life!

Dr. Doug Willen can be reached at drdoug@The-HealthFixer.com

Because of the demands of practicing full-time, lecturing, writing, and maintaining two blogs and numerous video projects, I cannot answer medical questions unless you are a patient. I will respond to as many e-mails as possible that are not medically oriented in content. I am always open to hearing about results and success stories; include whether you want your success stories to be in the blog or future books, and how you want your name to appear. Depending on whether there is an interest or not, I may have a Private Memberhip Area on the PaleoSoul.com site where you can post your questions and check back for answers. The Q & A will be handled in an open forum. This area will have a low monthly fee. Look for this area of the website to be functional in the fall of 2012.

Dr. Doug's Websites:
The hub or introduction page is at DougWillen.com

1.   TheHealthFixer.com

"This website has info on Dr. Doug Willen's NYC practice called Willen Wellness. This is also Dr. Doug's original blog about natural solutions to common health concerns. Dr. Willen shares stories and cases from his everyday practice in NYC with his diverse patient base. Learn how to visit Willen Wellness for expert nutritional and chiropractic care. Information on booking a phone consultation with Dr. Doug is located on this site"

2.   PaleoSoul.com

"Dr. Doug Willen writes with heart and 15 years of clinical experience behind him, on great nutrition, health, successful weight loss and the personal transformation required to realize and maintain these goals. His passion connects you to the science, body and soul of the Paleo lifestyle."

3.   QuantumPaleo.com

Quantum Paleo, a super-result-producing program is available to individuals through our Webinar series (coming fall of 2012), private one-on-one coaching with Dr. Doug, and as a dynamic corporate team-building competition that you can bring to your company. Dr. Doug also does a short format (3-4 hours) hands-on workshop for CrossFit Gym affiliates, major health clubs, and assorted community groups and businesses.

4.   PaleoXFit.com

"A 90-day body transformation documented on film. Dr. Doug 'walks the walk' and follows a strict Paleo Diet while training 3-4 days per week at CrossFit Hell's Kitchen. Ten segments track the ups and downs."

Websites to know on Paleolithic stuff:

RobbWolf.com   Robb Wolf, an expert in Paleolithic Nutrition. Fun, informative, a must.

MarksDailyApple.com

> This is Mark Sisson's site. He has the largest Paleo/Primal site on the Internet.

ThePaleoDiet.com

> Dr. Loren Cordain's ground-breaking book and website. Many people think of him as the leading expert in the world on the Paleo Diet. He was certainly the first to hit the scene and write the first best-selling book in this arena.

Whole9Life.com

> Great site, to learn, and get inspired. This couple walks the walk, and delivers great info.

Archevore.com

> Kurt Harris, M.D., I love his articles, comments and rants.

EatWild.com

> More food info on wild food sources.

GrasslandBeef.com

> An online store selling grass-fed beef, lamb, chicken, pork, bison, wild seafood, rabbit, and other Paleo goodies.

http://www.montereybayaquarium.org/cr/seafood-watch.aspx

> This site posts the dos and don'ts for buying seafood that is safe and sustainable

http://drcate.com   Dr. Cate Shanahan's health and wellness site.

Cookbooks

1 *Paleo Cookbook- Complete Paleo Recipe Guide to healthy eating!*
(Ebook at PaleoSoul.com or PaleoXFit.com)

2 *Primal Blueprint Cookbook* by Mark Sisson

3 *Everyday Paleo* by Sarah Fragoso

4 *The Paleo Diet Cookbook* by Loren Cordain

Great Reads

The Paleo Diet by Loren Cordain

The Paleo Solution by Robb Wolf

Wheat Belly by William Davis, M.D.

Why We Get Fat by Gary Taubes

Dangerous Grains by Braly and Hoggan

Primal Blueprint by Mark Sisson

Primal Body, Primal Mind by Nora T. Gedgaudas

Pandora's Seed by Spencer Wells

CrossFit

http://CrossFit.com

Here is a youtube video that shows CrossFit in action!

http://www.youtube.com/watch?v=tzD9BkXGJ1M ("What is CrossFit?")

Workshops:

Dr. Doug is available to teach *Quantum Paleo* workshops at CrossFit Gyms, Health Clubs, and other venues. He does corporate training and team building competitions on the topic of getting fit and staying well.

Be a part of the community! Sign-up for updates and free videos at either one of Dr. Doug's blogs!

TheHealthFixer.com
PaleoSoul.com

Dr. Doug is releasing a short book called: *What is Paleo?*

Here is a 4 minute video that Dr. Doug made titled: *What is Paleo?*

http://www.youtube.com/watch?v=choKVxBsPTI

What is Paleo? is a scaled down version of Quantum Paleo. Under 50 pages. *What is Paleo?* is a what-you-need-to-know book for someone to get started with this life-changing program without the stories and motivation. A printed version will be available soon on Amazon. *What is Paleo?* will make a great give-a-way to have on counter tops in health food stores, health clubs, CrossFit boxes and healthcare offices. It will also make a great book to share with friends and family that "don't understand why you are going Paleo"!

Suport and Phone Consults (TheHealthFixer.com)
Get "Health Fixed":

Get privately coached by Dr. Doug Willen to lose weight and build your health to the highest level!

After filling out a Symptom Survey. Meet with Dr. Doug privately on the phone, Skype, or Skype Video. The first call will be 45 minutes. Follow-up calls are based on 5 minute time units. The average follow-up can be completed in 10-15 minutes. Go to http:// TheHealthFixer.com and click on the "Phone Consult" link for more information.

Start building your health immediately!

1   Natural solutions to your specific health issues.
2   Dr. Doug will recommend specific supplements, herbs, detox and homeopathic products that will target your specific health issues.
3   Custom designed paleo diet program monitored by Dr. Doug.

4 Build a health support program that will address: thyroid balance, adrenal fatigue, hormone balance, digestion, fatigue, auto-immune, blood sugar issues, chronic pain, inflammation, celiac, food and gluten intolerances, ADD, ADHD and more!

5 Decide on your weight loss goals and partner with Dr. Doug to make it a reality. Many people find that the "accountability" aspect is the missing factor!

Food Sensitivities and food Intolerances!

Find out your specific food intolerances thru lab testing. Dr. Doug has been doing IgG Food Sensitivity testing for 14 years. How would you like to know if dairy, egg, grains and 96 total foods are causing a delayed drain on your health and immune system. Go to TheHealthFixer.com and learn about this life-changing test.

Future Webinars:

Please send me feedback if you have interest in participating in a group class conducted thru an online Webinar format. This will be offered at a reduced price.

The Webinars will provide a way to participate from anywhere in the world directly with Dr. Doug.

Possible Webinar Topics:

A) *Quantum Paleo* 21-day Weight loss group

B) Natural Hormone Balance

C) How to conquer fatigue

D) Thyroid and Adrenal Balance

E) Eating for A's:

F) How to create a Health Miracle!

Let me know which topics you may be interested in. If I see an interest, I will start to put together a schedule of programs. (DrDoug@TheHealthFixer.com)

Social Media

I would love to stay in touch and learn more about your journey!

Connect with me thru:

Facebook: Facebook.com/DrDougWillen or
Facebook.com/TheHealthFixer

Twitter: Twitter.com/DrDougWillen

Bibliography

Andersen, H. C., Edgar Lucas, H. B. Paull, and Arthur Szyk. *Andersen's Fairy Tales*. New York: Grosset & Dunlap, 1945. Print.

Appleton, Nancy. *Lick the Sugar Habit*. Garden City Park, NY: Avery Pub. Group, 1996. Print.

Astrup, A., and J. Dyerberg. "The Role of Reducing Intakes of Saturated Fat in the Prevention of Cardiovascular Disease: Where Does the Evidence Stand in 2010." *Am Journal of Clinical Nutrition*. 4th ser. 93.April (2011): 684-8. Print.

Balch, Phyllis A., and James F. Balch. *Prescription for Nutritional Healing*. New York: Avery, 2000. Print.

Ballentine, Rudolph. *Diet and Nutrition a Holistic Approach*. Honesdale,Pa: Himalayan International Institute, 1979. Print.

Batmanghelidj, F. *Your Body's Many Cries for Water.*
[S.l.]: Tagman, 2004. Print.

Borhanihaghighi, A., N. Ansari, M. Mokhtari, B.
Geramizadeh, and K. Lankarani. "Multiple Sclerosis
and Gluten Sensitivity☆." *Clinical Neurology and
Neurosurgery.* 109.8 (2007): 651-53. Print.

Braly, James, and Ron Hoggan. *Dangerous Grains:
Why Gluten Cereal Grains May Be Hazardous to Your
Health.* New York: Avery, 2002. Print.

Briani, C., D. Samaroo, and A. Alaedini. "Celiac Disease: From Gluten to Autoimmunity." *Autoimmunity
Reviews.* 7.8 (2008): 644-50. Print.

Brody, Julia Green, Ruthann A. Rudel, Karin B. Mi-
chels, and Kirsten B. Moysich. "Environmental Pol-
lutants, Diet, Physical Activity, Body Size, and Breast
Cancer." *Cancer.* 109.S12 (2007): 2627-634. Print.

Case, Shelley. *Gluten-free Diet: A Comprehensive
Resource Guide.* Regina: Case Nutrition Consulting,
2002. Print.

Challem, Jack, Burt Berkson, and Melissa Diane.
Smith. *Syndrome X: The Complete Nutritional Pro-
gram to Prevent and Reverse Insulin Resistance.* New
York: Wiley, 2000. Print.

Chevat, Richie, and Michael Pollan. *The Omnivore's Dilemma: The Secrets behind What You Eat*. New York: Dial, 2009. Print.

Cohen, Mark Nathan. *Health and the Rise of Civilization*. New Haven: Yale UP, 1989. Print.

Collin, Pekka, and Timo Reunala. "Recognition and Management of the Cutaneous Manifestations of Celiac Disease." *American Journal of Clinical Dermatology*. 4.1 (2003): 13-20. Print.

Cordain, Loren. "Introduction." *The Paleo Diet: Lose Weight and Get Healthy by Eating the Food You Were Designed to Eat*. New York: Wiley, 2003. 3-7. Print.

Crawford, Michael A., Richard P. Bazinet, and Andrew J. Sinclair. "Fat Intake and CNS Functioning: Ageing and Disease." *Annals of Nutrition and Metabolism*. 55.1-3 (2009): 202-28. Print.

Crawford, Michael, and David Marsh. *The Nutrition and Evolution*. New Canaan, CT: Keats Publ., 1995. Print.

Croft, N. "IgG Food Antibodies and Irritating the Bowel." *Gastroenterology*. 128.4 (2005): 1135-136. Print.

Davis, William, and John A. Rumberger. *Track Your Plaque: The Only Heart Disease Prevention Program That Shows You How to Use the New Heart Scans to Detect, Track, and Control Coronary Plaque*. New York: IUniverse, 2004. Print.

De Lorgeril, Michel, Patricia Salen, Jean-Louis Martin, François Boucher, and Joël De Leiris. "Interactions of Wine Drinking with Omega-3 Fatty Acids in Patients with Coronary Heart Disease: A Fish-like Effect of Moderate Wine Drinking." *American Heart Journal*. 155.1 (2008): 175-81. Print.

Della Valle, N., S. Prencipe, and V. De Francesco. "P.208 Body Composition And Dietary Intakes In Adult Coeliac Disease Patients From Southern Italy Consuming A Strict Gluten-Free Diet." *Digestive and Liver Disease*. 42 (2010): S175. Print.

Diamond, Jared M. *The Third Chimpanzee: The Evolution and Future of the Human Animal*. New York: HarperPerennial, 2006. Print.

Dickey, William, and Natalie Kearney. "Overweight in Celiac Disease: Prevalence, Clinical Characteristics, and Effect of a Gluten-Free Diet." The *American Journal of Gastroenterology*. 101.10 (2006): 2356-359. Print.

Docena, G. H., R. Fernandez, F. G. Chirdo, and C. A. Fossati. "Identification of Casein as the Major Allergenic and Antigenic Protein of Cow's Milk." *Allergy*. 51.6 (1996): 412-16. Print.

Donnelly, Joseph E., Bryan Smith, Dennis J. Jacobsen, Erik Kirk, Katrina DuBose, Melissa Hyder, Bruce Bailey, and Richard Washburn. "The Role of Exercise for Weight Loss and Maintenance." *Best Practice & Research Clinical Gastroenterology*. 18.6 (2004): 1009-029. Print.

Dorland, W. A. Newman. *Dorland's Medical Dictionary*. Philadelphia, PA: Saunders, 1980. Print.

Eades, Michael R., and Mary Dan. Eades. *Protein Power: The High Protein, Low Carbohydrate Way to Lose Weight, Feel Fit, and Boost Your Health*. London: Thorsons, 2000. Print.

Eades, Michael R., and Mary Dan. Eades. *Protein Power: The Metabolic Breakthrough*. New York: Bantam, 1996. Print.

Eaton, S.Boyd, and Melvin Konner. "Paleolithic Nutrition." *The New England Journal of Medicine*. 312. (5) (1985): 283-89. Print.

Elder, Jennifer Harrison, Meena Shankar, and Jonathan Shuster. "The Gluten-Free, Casein-Free Diet In Autism: Results of A Preliminary Double Blind Clinical Trial." *Journal of Autism and Developmental*

Disorders. 36.3 (2006): 413-20. Print.

"The Emperor's New Clothes." *Wikipedia.* Web. 30 Dec. 2011. <http://en.wikipedia.org/wiki/The_Emperor's_New_Clothes>.

Enig, Mary G. *Know Your Fats: The Complete Primer for Understanding the Nutrition of Fats, Oils and Cholesterol.* Silver Spring, MD: Bethesda, 2000. Print.

Erasmus, Udo. *Fats That Heal, Fats That Kill: The Complete Guide to Fats, Oils, Cholesterol, and Human Health.* Burnaby, BC, Canada: Alive, 1993. Print.

Frost, Robert. *Mountain Interval.* New York: H. Holt and, 1921. Print.

Fuehrlein, B. S. "Differential Metabolic Effects of Saturated Versus Polyunsaturated Fats in Ketogenic Diets." *Journal of Clinical Endocrinology & Metabolism.* 89.4 (2004): 1641-645. Print.

Gannon, M. C., and F. Q. Nuttall. "Effect of a High-Protein, Low-Carbohydrate Diet on Blood Glucose Control in People With Type 2 Diabetes." *Diabetes.* 53.9 (2004): 2375-382. Print.

Gittleman, Ann Louise. *The Fat Flush Plan.* New York: McGraw-Hill, 2002. Print.

Glassman, Greg. "Nutrition: An Interview With Fast Company Magazine." *CrossFit Journal*. Fast Track Magazine Exclusive Interview, 11 Oct. 2011. Web. <http://journal.crossfit.com/2011/10/greggamesnutrition.tpl>.

Goldfinger, T. "Beyond the French Paradox: The Impact of Moderate Beverage Alcohol and Wine Consumption in the Prevention of Cardiovascular Disease." *Cardiology Clinics*. 21.3 (2003): 449-57. Print.

Guyton, Arthur C., and John E. Hall. *Textbook of Medical Physiology*. Philadelphia: Saunders, 2000. Print.

Hadjivassiliou, Marios, David S. Sanders, Richard A. Grünewald, Nicola Woodroofe, Sabrina Boscolo, and Daniel Aeschlimann. "Gluten Sensitivity: From Gut to Brain." *The Lancet Neurology*. 9.3 (2010): 318-30. Print.

Hays, J. H. "The Hunter-Gatherer Diet." *Mayo Clinic Proceedings*. 79 (5) May (2004): 703-04. Print.

Heaton, K. "Sugar Consumption And Myocardial Infarction." *The Lancet*. 297.7691 (1971): 185-86. Print.

Hill, Napoleon. *Think and Grow Rich*. North Hollywood, CA: Wilshire Book, 1966. Print.

Horne, J. "Obesity and Short Sleep: Unlikely Bedfellows?" *Obesity Reviews* .(2011): No. Print.

Hunt, Charles. *Charles Hunt's Diet Evolution: Eat Fat and Get Fit!*. Beverly Hills, CA: Maximum Human Potential Productions, 1999. Print.

Hutchinson, Ezzie. "Celiac Disease: Increased Celiac Disease in IBS." *Nature Reviews Gastroenterology & Hepatology.* 6.7 (2009): 381. Print.

Ivy, John L. "Role of Exercise Training in the Prevention and Treatment of Insulin Resistance and Non-Insulin-Dependent Diabetes Mellitus." *Sports Medicine.* 24.5 (1997): 321-36. Print.

Kalaydjian, A. E., W. Eaton, N. Cascella, and A. Fasano. "The Gluten Connection: The Association between Schizophrenia and Celiac Disease." *Acta Psychiatrica Scandinavica.* 113.2 (2006): 82-90. Print.

Kaufmann, Doug A., and Beverly Thornhill. Hunt. *The Fungus Link: An Introduction to Fungal Disease including the Initial Phase Diet.* Rockwall, TX: MediaTrition, 2000. Print.

Kaufmann, Doug A., and Beverly Thornhill. Hunt. *The Germ That Causes Cancer: With the Initial Phase Diet, Cancer Edition.* Rockwall, TX: MediaTrition, 2002. Print.

Kaufmann, Doug A., and David Holland. *What Makes Bread Rise?: A Science-based Weight Loss Program for America's Families*. Rockwall, TX: MediaTrition, 2004. Print.

Lee, Richard B., and Richard Heywood Daly. *The Cambridge Encyclopedia of Hunters and Gatherers*. Cambridge, U.K.: Cambridge UP, 1999. Print.

Lefebvre, and Scheen. "Glucose Metabolism and the Postprandial State." *European Journal of Clinical Investigation*. 29.S2 (1999): 1-6. Print.

Lieberman, Shari, and Linda Segall. *The Gluten Connection: How Gluten Sensitivity May Be Sabotaging Your Health-- and What You Can Do to Take Control Now*. [Emmaus, Penn.]: Rodale, 2007. Print.

Lipski, Elizabeth. *Digestive Wellness: Strengthen the Immune System and Prevent Disease through Healthy Digestion*. New York, NY: McGraw-Hill, 2012. Print.

Liska, DeAnn, and Jeffrey Bland. *Clinical Nutrition: A Functional Approach*. Gig Harbor, WA: Institute for Functional Medicine, 2004. Print.

Lorenzen, J. "Gluten-Sensitive Enteropathy And Eczema." *The Lancet*. 285.7388 (1965): 766. Print.

Ludwig, D., K. Peterson, and S. Gortmaker. "Relation

between Consumption of Sugar-sweetened Drinks and Childhood Obesity: A Prospective, Observational Analysis." *The Lancet.* 357.9255 (2001): 505-08. Print.

Marshall, N., N. Glozier, and R. Grunstein. "Is Sleep Duration Related to Obesity? A Critical Review of the Epidemiological Evidence." *Sleep Medicine Reviews.* 12.4 (2008): 289-98. Print.

McClenaghan, Neville H. "Determining the Relationship between Dietary Carbohydrate Intake and Insulin Resistance." *Nutrition Research Reviews.* 18.02 (2005): 222. Print.

Melanson, Edward L., Arne Astrup, and William T. Donahoo. "The Relationship between Dietary Fat and Fatty Acid Intake and Body Weight, Diabetes, and the Metabolic Syndrome." *Annals of Nutrition and Metabolism.* 55.1-3 (2009): 229-43. Print.

Melnik, Bodo C. "Milk – The Promoter of Chronic Western Diseases." *Medical Hypotheses.* 72.6 (2009): 631-39. Print.

Moneret Vautrin, D. A., J. Sainte-Laudy, and G. Kanny. "Ulcerative Colitis Possibly Due to Hypersensitivity to Wheat and Egg." *Allergy.* 56.5 (2001): 458-59. Print.

Niewinski, M. "Advances in Celiac Disease and Gluten-Free Diet." *Journal of the American Dietetic Association.* 108.4 (2008): 661-72. Print.

Null, Gary. *Nutrition and the Mind.* New York: Four Walls Eight Windows, 1995. Print.

"Nutrition, Insulin, Insulin-like Growth Factors and Cancer." *Hormone and Metabolic Research.* 35.11/12 (2003): 694-704. Print.

Parker, G., N. A. Gibson, H. Brotchie, G. Heruc, A.-M. Rees, and D. Hadzi-Pavlovic. "Omega-3 Fatty Acids and Mood Disorders." *American Journal of Psychiatry.* 163.6 (2006): 969-78. Print.

Patel, Sanjay R., and Frank B. Hu. "Short Sleep Duration and Weight Gain: A Systematic Review." *Obesity.* 16.3 (2008): 643-53. Print.

Percheron, C. "Metabolic Responses to High Carbohydrate Breakfasts in Obese Patients with Impaired Glucose Tolerance. Comparison of Meals Containing Dairy Products and Fruits versus Bread." *Nutrition Research.* 17.5 (1997): 797-806. Print.

Pert, Candace B. *Molecules of Emotion.* New York: Scribner, 2003. Print.

Peskin, Brian, and Marcus Conyers. *Beyond the Zone.* Houston, TX: Noble Pub., 2000. Print.

"Phytate And Rickets." *Nutrition Reviews.* 31.8 (1973): 238-39. Print.

Pottenger, Francis M., Elaine Pottenger, and Robert T. Pottenger. *Pottenger's Cats: A Study in Nutrition.* La Mesa, CA (P.O. Box 2614, La Mesa 92041): Price-Pottenger Nutrition Foundation, 2009. Print.

Price, Weston. *Nutrition and Physical Degeneration: A Comparison of Primitive and Modern Diets and Their Effects.* (Hardback). Garsington: Benediction Classics, 2010. Print.

Ray, Sondra. *The Only Diet There Is.* Berkeley, CA: Celestial Arts, 1981. Print.

Rippetoe, Mark, and Lon Kilgore. *Starting Strength: Basic Barbell Training.* Wichita Falls, TX: Aasgaard, 2007. Print.

Robinson, Jo. *Pasture Perfect: The Far-reaching Benefits of Choosing Meat, Eggs, and Dairy Products from Grass-fed Animals.* Vashon, WA: Vashon Island, 2004. Print.

Ross, Julia. *The Mood Cure: The 4-step Program to Rebalance Your Emotional Chemistry and Rediscover*

Your Natural Sense of Well-being. New York: Viking, 2002. Print.

Rozynek, P., and I. Sander. "TPIS - an IgE-binding Wheat Protein." *Allergy.* 57.5 (2002): 463. Print.

Ryan, Alice S. "Exercise in Aging: Its Important Role in Mortality, Obesity and Insulin Resistance." *Aging Health.* 6.5 (2010): 551-63. Print.

Ryan, Frank. *The Eskimo Diet: How to Avoid a Heart Attack.* Ebury Press, 1990. Print.

Schmid, Ronald F. *The Untold Story of Milk: The History, Politics and Science of Nature's Perfect Food : Raw Milk from Pasture-fed Cows.* Washington, DC: NewTrends Pub., 2009. Print.

Sears, Barry. *The Zone.* New York: HarperCollins, 1995. Print.

Shakespeare, William. *Romeo and Juliet.* Act II.,Sc. II ed. Oxford,Eng.: Oxford UP., 2002. Print.

Simopoulos, A. P. "Omega 3 Fatty Acids in the Prevention-management of Cardiovascular Disease." *Can J Physiol Pharmacol.* 1997.75 (1997): 234-9. Print.

Sinatra, Stephen T., James Roberts, and Martin

Zucker. *Reverse Heart Disease Now: Stop Deadly Cardiovascular Plaque before It's Too Late.* Hoboken, NJ: John Wiley & Sons, 2007. Print.

Sivak, M. "Sleeping More as a Way to Lose Weight." *Obesity Reviews* 7.3 (2006): 295-96. Print.

Soleas, George J., Eleftherios P. Diamandis, and David M. Goldberg. "Wine as a Biological Fluid: History, Production, and Role in Disease Prevention." *Journal of Clinical Laboratory Analysis.* 11.5 (1997): 287-313. Print.

Speth, John D. "Early Hominid Hunting and Scavenging: The Role of Meat as an Energy Source." *Journal of Human Evolution.* 18.4 (1989): 329-43. Print.

Spiegel, K. "Sleep Loss: A Novel Risk Factor for Insulin Resistance and Type 2 Diabetes." Journal of Applied Physiology 99.5 (2005): 2008-019. Print.

Stanford, Craig B. *The Hunting Apes: Meat Eating and the Origins of Human Behavior.* Princeton, NJ: Princeton UP, 1999. Print.

Stockman, J.a. "The Effects of Low-Carbohydrate Versus Conventional Weight Loss Diets in Severely Obese Adults: One-Year Follow-up of a Randomized Trial." *Yearbook of Pediatrics.* 2006 (2006): 428-31. Print.

Tatham, A. S., and P. R. Shewry. "Allergy to Wheat and Related Cereals." *Clinical & Experimental Allergy.* (2008). Print.

Tau, C., C. Mautalen, and S. De Rosa. "Bone Mineral Density in Children with Celiac Disease. Effect of a Gluten-free Diet." *European Journal of Clinical Nutrition.* 60.3 (2005): 358-63. Print.

Tsatsouline, Pavel. *The Naked Warrior: Master the Secrets of the Super-strong, Using Bodyweight Exercises Only.* St. Paul, MN: Dragon Door, 2004. Print.

Van Cauter, E., and K. L. Knutson. "Sleep and the Epidemic of Obesity in Children and Adults." *European Journal of Endocrinology.* 159.Suppl_1 (2008): S59-66. Print.

Walford, Roy L. *The 120-year Diet: How to Double Your Vital Years.* New York: Simon and Schuster, 1986. Print.

Werlinger, Kelly, Teresa K. King, Matthew M. Clark, Vincent Pera, and John P. Wincze. "Perceived Changes in Sexual Functioning and Body Image following Weight Loss in an Obese Female Population: A Pilot Study." *Journal of Sex & Marital Therapy.* 23.1 (1997): 74-78. Print.

Wilson, James L. *Adrenal Fatigue: The 21st Century Stress Syndrome.* Petaluma, CA: Smart Publications, 2001. Print.

Wolf, Robb. *The Paleo Solution: The Original Human Diet.* Las Vegas: Victory Belt, 2010. Print.

Zimmet, P., and C. R. Thomas. "Genotype, Obesity, and Cardiovascular Disease: Has Technical and Social Advancement Outstripped Evolution?" *Journal of Internal Medicine.* 2nd ser. Aug.254 (2003): 114-25. Print.

Zipes, Jack. *Hans Christian Andersen: The Misunderstood Storyteller.* New York: Routledge, 2005. Print.

CPSIA information can be obtained at www.ICGtesting.com
Printed in the USA
BVOW020152211112

306082BV00001B/2/P